A Look Back:
The Birth
of the Americans
with Disabilities Act

A Look Back: The Birth of the Americans with Disabilities Act

Robert C. Anderson, MDiv
Editor

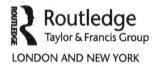

Routledge
Taylor & Francis Group

LONDON AND NEW YORK

First published 1996 by The Haworth Press, Inc.

2 Park Square, Milton Park, Abingdon, Oxon OX14 4RN
605 Third Avenue, New York, NY 10017

Routledge is an imprint of the Taylor & Francis Group, an informa business

A Look Back: The Birth of the Americans with Disabilities Act has also been published as *Journal of Religion in Disability & Rehabilitation*, Volume 2, Number 4 1996.

First issued in paperback 2022

Library of Congress Cataloging-in-Publication Data

A look back : the birth of the Americans with Disabilities Act / Robert C. Anderson, editor.
     p. cm.
     Includes bibliographical references.
     ISBN 0-7890-0007-5 (alk. paper)
     1. Handicapped–Civil rights–United States. 2. Church work with the handicapped–United States. 3. Handicapped–Religious aspects–Christianity. 4. Discrimination against the handicapped–Law and legislation–United States. 5. United States. Americans with Disabilities Act of 1990. I. Anderson, Robert C. (Robert Carl), 1961- .
HV1553.L66 1996
323.3'087–dc20   96-19551
                                                       CIP

ISBN 13: 978-0-789-00007-1 (hbk)
ISBN 13: 978-1-03-234040-1 (pbk)
DOI: 10.4324/9781315862514

This book is dedicated to **The Reverend Harold H. Wilke, DD**
Pioneer advocate in the field of Religion and Disability

A Look Back:
The Birth of the Americans
with Disabilities Act

CONTENTS

ABOUT THE EDITOR

Robert C. Anderson, MDiv, is Director of the Lakeshore Foundation's Religion and Disability Program (Birmingham, Alabama). The program is a state-based community model which assists congregations in their efforts to become more welcoming and inclusive to persons with disabilities.

Reverend Anderson received his Master of Divinity in Pastoral Care and Counseling at the Southern Baptist Theological Seminary in Louisville, Kentucky and his Clinical Pastoral Education residency at the Cathedral Church of the Advent (Episcopal) in Birmingham, Alabama. Before joining the Lakeshore Foundation, he served for six years as Chaplain at Lakeshore Rehabilitation Hospital. His practical and research interests include helping persons with disabilities form and maintain connections to the community, particularly through local congregations.

Reverend Anderson works primarily with congregations and communities at the local level, although he is available to offer assistance statewide. He serves on the board of directors for the Alabama Coalition of Citizens with Disabilities and the Birmingham Independent Living Center. He also consults with the *Spiritual Care in Rehabilitation* Task Force of the American Congress of Rehabilitation Medicine. Reverend Anderson writes and speaks in the field of religion and disability.

Introductory Note from the Office of Former President George Bush

One of my proudest moments as President occurred on July 26, 1990—the day I signed the Americans with Disabilities Act into law (see Photograph 1). With its passage, a shameful wall of exclusion came tumbling down. This landmark legislation was the culmination of the dedicated efforts of so many, and I salute the bipartisan leadership of the Congress—as well as the countless advocates from all parts of society who contributed to our success. It was a team effort.

With the ADA, our country took a dramatic step toward eliminating the physical barriers that existed and the social barriers that were accepted. Much work lies ahead, but I am confident that we will finish the wonderful work already begun. After all, it's the right thing to do.

The Honorable George Bush

[Haworth co-indexing entry note]: "Introductory Note from the Office of Former President George Bush." Bush, George. Co-published simultaneously in *Journal of Religion in Disability & Rehabilitation* (The Haworth Press, Inc.) Vol. 2, No. 4, 1996, pp. 1-2; and: *A Look Back: The Birth of the Americans with Disabilities Act* (ed: Robert C. Anderson) The Haworth Press, Inc., 1996, pp. 1-2. Single or multiple copies of this article are available from The Haworth Document Delivery Service [1-800-342-9678, 9:00 a.m. - 5:00 p.m. (EST). E-mail address: getinfo@haworth.com].

PHOTOGRAPH 1. Signing of the Americans with Disabilities Act, July 26, 1990, South Lawn, The White House. HIS LEFT FOOT—The Reverend Harold Wilke of Claremont, California accepts the pen from President George Bush with his left foot after the president signed the Act into law. Reverend Wilke has no arms and uses his feet for hands. Vice President Dan Quayle, left, and Evan Kemp, in wheelchair (former chairman of the Equal Employment Opportunity Commission) look on.

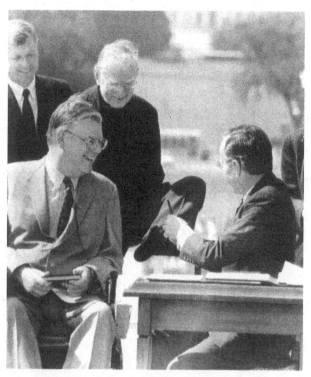

Photo Courtesy AP/WideWorld Photo. Used by permission.
Publication usage fee paid by the Lakeshore Foundation, Birmingham, Alabama.

To Rev. Harold Wilke
Thank you for blessing this special, historic event
Sincerely, Geo Bush

Blessing:
Delivered at the Presidential Signing
of the Americans with Disabilities Act

"Let my people go!" was your decree, O God,
Commanding that all your children be freed from the bonds of slavery.

Today we celebrate the breaking of the chains which have held back millions of Americans with disabilities.

Today we celebrate the granting to them of full citizenship and access to the Promised Land of work, service and community.

Bless this gathering . . . this joyous celebration.

Bless our President as he signs the Americans with Disabilities Act. Strengthen our resolve as we take up the task, knowing that our work has just begun.

Bless the American people and move them to discard those old beliefs and attitudes that limit and diminish those among us with disabilities.

Our prayer is in your name, O God, whom we call by many names: the God and Father of our Lord Jesus Christ; Allah, the Compassionate and Merciful One; the God of Abraham, Isaac and Jacob and of Rebeccah and Sarah and Ruth; the Ground of all Being, the Infinite Source of Love and Light.

Amen.

The Reverend Harold H. Wilke, DD
South Lawn, The White House
July 26, 1990

[Haworth co-indexing entry note]: "Blessing: Delivered at the Presidential Signing of the Americans with Disabilities Act." Wilke, Harold H. Co-published simultaneously in *Journal of Religion in Disability & Rehabilitation* (The Haworth Press, Inc.) Vol. 2, No. 4, 1996, p. 3; and: *A Look Back: The Birth of the Americans with Disabilities Act* (ed: Robert C. Anderson) The Haworth Press, Inc., 1996, p. 3. Single or multiple copies of this article are available from The Haworth Document Delivery Service [1-800-342-9678, 9:00 a.m. - 5:00 p.m. (EST). E-mail address: getinfo@haworth.com].

Tribute to an Advocate:
Harold H. Wilke, DD

Alan A. Reich, MA, MBA

SUMMARY. The author offers personal and professional affirmation about the career of one of this century's most esteemed statesmen in religion and disability. *[Article copies available from The Haworth Document Delivery Service: 1-800-342-9678. E-mail address: getinfo@haworth.com]*

KEYWORDS. Advocate, disability, ADA, Americans with Disabilities Act, Wilke

Reverend Harold H. Wilke's sermon, "The All Embracing Arms," delivered recently at the New York Avenue Presbyterian Church in Washington, is particularly poignant when one remembers that he has no arms. His theme of *encapsulating grace* educated us all about the true gifts of those with disabilities.

Equally marvelous to me is Harold's undaunted spirit, so much in evidence when I drove him to the airport that afternoon for his return home to California. No one was available to assist with his bag. Unperturbed, Harold opened the car door with his left foot.

Alan A. Reich is President of the National Organization on Disability in Washington, DC. He received his Diploma in Slavonic Studies from Oxford University and his MBA from Harvard University.

[Haworth co-indexing entry note]: "Tribute to an Advocate: Harold H. Wilke, DD." Reich, Alan A. Co-published simultaneously in *Journal of Religion in Disability & Rehabilitation* (The Haworth Press, Inc.) Vol. 2, No. 4, 1996, pp. 5-7; and: *A Look Back: The Birth of the Americans with Disabilities Act* (ed: Robert C. Anderson) The Haworth Press, Inc., 1996, pp. 5-7. Single or multiple copies of this article are available from The Haworth Document Delivery Service [1-800-342-9678, 9:00 a.m. - 5:00 p.m. (EST). E-mail address: getinfo@haworth.com].

When I asked about the bag, he said, "Don't worry, Alan. I'll carry it with my teeth." (He declined my proposal to have him remove my wheelchair from the car trunk with his teeth so that I could carry his bag on my lap.) As I drove off, Harold and the bag were already inside the terminal. He'd slung it over his shoulder with the left foot. All in a day's work for the Reverend Harold Wilke!

Harold Wilke is a truly amazing man: author, scholar, teacher; motivational speaker, activist, visionary; role model, clergyman, parent; world leader and friend. These are just a few of the words that come to mind when I think of Harold. I first met him in 1982 when I was heading up the International Year of Disabled Persons (IYDP) for the United Nations. Harold was already world renowned as a religious leader and disability advocate. But nothing I heard prepared me for meeting him that first time.

I can still remember the look of wonder on the faces of the IYDP Council staff as Harold stood to address them. He pulled a pen out of his breast pocket, removed the top, then took out a business card, signed and presented it to a stunned staff member. Harold did it all (graciously and tastefully) with his foot!

Harold has never let his disability get in the way of his abundant, God-given talents and ability. He learned early that no challenge is so great that it can't be overcome with dedication, hard work and a sense of humor.

Harold was one of the first disability leaders to speak out on behalf of the 500 million people with disabilities in the world. As leader of the People-to-People Committee of Persons with Disabilities in the 1970s, he traveled extensively around the globe, promoting the message of hope for all people with disabilities.

Although he is one of the most cooperative members of any group, Harold is not afraid to "march to the beat of his own drum," particularly after conferring with the Almighty. His speech to the Vatican Conference on Disability Worldwide in 1992 is a memorable example of his independent thinking and strong faith. As a member of the World Committee, Harold had (as requested) submitted his prepared remarks on the caring congregation long beforehand to the Vatican. Nine thousand interfaith delegates gathered in the Vatican's great Victor Emmanuel Hall. Before that great assembly, Harold put aside his prepared text and spoke extemporaneously about the gifts each man and woman brings to the caring congregation. Pope John Paul II who came to the conference the next day and specifically sought out Harold, embracing him and thanking him for his lifelong commitment to the spiritual well-being of all people, everywhere.

Harold is a founding director of the National Organization on Disability (NOD), endowing it with a rich legacy. In 1985, Harold noted that religion and spiritual life are very important to persons with disabilities and urged NOD to develop a national Religion and Disability program. The board unanimously agreed.

Three years later, Harold found the ideal person in Ginny Thornburgh to direct NOD's interfaith outreach efforts. Since then Ginny, along with Harold as her mentor, has co-authored two popular guides: *That All May Worship* and *Loving Justice,* which have helped thousands of congregations to be more accessible and welcoming to persons with disabilities.

In 1990, Harold played a unique role in an historic ceremony that took place on the south lawn of the White House. On that hot July 26th day, Harold stood next to President George Bush and gave a blessing before the signing of the Americans with Disabilities Act (ADA), the most significant civil rights legislation in recent decades.

We believe this to be the first time in our nation's history that a blessing accompanied a presidential bill signing. It was only appropriate that Reverend Harold H. Wilke, disability rights pioneer whose ministry embraces the world, was the person chosen to lead those assembled in prayer.

At 80 years of age, Harold is still going strong, speaking to congregations and community groups around the country, writing articles, teaching, encouraging seminaries to include disability within their curricula, and by being pastor and mentor to so many.

Through his enthusiasm, self-acceptance, grit and twinkle, he reminds us that every person (with or without a disability) has unique gifts to offer. The Reverend Harold Wilke's life and work bear testimony that one man can indeed make an enormous difference in the world.

The Significance
of the ADA to All Americans:
The Process of Getting It,
and Now That We Have It,
How Is It Shaping Up?

Evan J. Kemp, Jr., JD

SUMMARY. The author provides background information about the Americans with Disabilities Act's development. His involvement with the Equal Employment Opportunity Commission during the Bush Administration adds insight, along with his personal experience with disability. The discussion includes a look at both sides of this landmark legislation. *[Article copies available from The Haworth Document Delivery Service: 1-800-342-9678. E-mail address: getinfo@haworth.com]*

KEYWORDS. Americans with Disabilities Act, ADA, disability, advocacy

Before the Americans with Disabilities Act (ADA) was adopted, the primary legislation that prohibited discrimination against people

---

The Honorable Evan J. Kemp, Jr., is the former Chairman of the Equal Employment Opportunity Commission, a wheelchair driver, and a disability rights advocate for the past 30 years. He is presently Senior Partner in the communications and marketing firm of Evan Kemp Associates, Washington, DC.

[Haworth co-indexing entry note]: "The Significance of the ADA to All Americans: The Process of Getting It, and Now That We Have It, How Is It Shaping Up?" Kemp, Evan J., Jr. Co-published simultaneously in *Journal of Religion in Disability & Rehabilitation* (The Haworth Press, Inc.) Vol. 2, No. 4, 1996, pp. 9-14; and: *A Look Back: The Birth of the Americans with Disabilities Act* (ed: Robert C. Anderson) The Haworth Press, Inc., 1996, pp. 9-14. Single or multiple copies of this article are available from The Haworth Document Delivery Service [1-800-342-9678, 9:00 a.m. - 5:00 p.m. (EST). E-mail address: getinfo@haworth.com].

with disabilities was sections 503 and 504 of the Rehabilitation Act of 1973. However, this protection was only available through entities that received any type of federal funding. Businesses, public facilities, and other private organizations that did not receive federal funding were not obligated to comply with the directives of sections 503 or 504.

Due to these limitations, it became clear that there was a need for legislation that provided a clear and comprehensive mandate to eliminate discrimination against all individuals with disabilities.

However, the need for this type of comprehensive legislation met substantial opposition. Both large and small businesses feared that the passage of these laws would significantly reduce their profits. Further, the cost of compliance and potential litigation might result in bankruptcy for many companies. Speculation about soaring increases in the cost of liability and health insurance emerged as a significant concern. State and local governments fretted that taxes would need to be increased to cover the cost of carrying out the law. Disability interest groups also worried that their issues would not be adequately incorporated into the final version of the proposed legislation.

Despite these difficulties, disability groups and related organizations developed a unified voice in presenting these issues to both sides of Congress. The Americans with Disabilities Act would have never become landmark legislation without the unified position of these disability groups—and bold government leadership. For example, people with visual impairments and those with hearing impairments joined forces to assure their inclusion under the ADA. Issues faced by the hearing impaired were being supported by those with mobility impairments. Linkages were established among many other disability groups and served to forge the powerful and unified voice of action necessary to push the ADA bill forward. As a result, the diverse groups of people with disabilities produced a cohesiveness that had never before existed.

July 26, 1990. Finally, the legislation was passed. Over 3,000 crowded the White House lawn to witness President Bush sign the ADA into law. More persons were present at the ADA's signing than at any previous enactment of legislation. This attendance record has not been broken and probably never will. People came because of the years of struggle and commitment that it took to make the freedom of equal access a civil right for 49 million Americans.

Most shared the feeling that life would be better now, not only for those who had persevered through the political hurdles of getting the ADA passed, but also for persons with disabilities for generations to come. Living without discrimination was possible because now, for the first time, people with disabilities had civil rights. These gains included rights to compete in the marketplace, to be considered for jobs based on one's ability, to use private and public transportation, and to enter buildings without barriers. It was indeed the beginning of a new era.

But the real work had just begun. Getting the ADA passed into law was one thing. Enforcement was an entirely different matter. The ADA's passage did not guarantee that discrimination in the work place would stop, or that every new building or facility would become accessible.

Some businesses decide not to voluntarily comply with accessibility requirements of the ADA, choosing to wait until they are taken to court. Others remain uninformed about the ADA altogether, while many think that it does not apply to them. Some employers take similar positions in matters concerning the equal employment opportunity provisions of the ADA.

Not only is the public unclear about the provisions of the ADA, so are the majority of people with disabilities. An estimated 70 percent are uninformed about their rights under the ADA. Educating the American people about their rights, obligations, responsibilities and protection under the ADA is essential for its implementation. Several federal programs provide grants to regional and state organizations to provide technical assistance and ADA training activities for businesses, state and local governments, and people with disabilities at the grass roots level. Getting word out through the various disability networks has reached a wide cross section of people with disabilities in the past five years. The challenge rests in contacting those who have not been associated with disability organizations. In addition to the grassroots approach, media awareness campaigns have reached many people who might not otherwise know about the provisions of the law.

IMPACT OF THE ADA FOR AMERICANS WITH DISABILITIES—SIX YEARS AFTER ITS PASSAGE

As transportation systems have become more accessible (and available), people with disabilities are able to participate in the community as much as they choose. Access standards for buildings and public facilities make it possible to get in the door of establishments that were previously inaccessible. The ADA's nondiscriminatory provisions afford people with disabilities more of an equal footing with others competing for the same job. Public schools have larger enrollments of students with disabilities because students have a chance at employment after graduation. With opportunity comes involvement—and visibility. For example, people with disabilities are more frequently seen on television programs and commercials, in political arenas, and at organized sports events. This was not the case 10 years ago. The ADA has played a major role in the process of people with disabilities having the same choices for leading independent lives as everyone else.

When it comes to enforcement, the provisions of the ADA are being challenged in the courts. Law firms and attorneys now take on steadily increasing numbers of ADA civil rights cases. A big part of the enforcement issue is cost. Most people with disabilities can't afford an attorney and aren't able to follow through in the courts. However, there are attorneys who take ADA cases on a pro bono basis or at reduced fees. Another concern is the lengthy process of having the matter addressed in the court system. As a result, mediation has emerged as a real alternative to resolving situations that would otherwise be costly and time consuming for all parties.

Several reports in the media have focused on criticisms of the ADA and perpetuate several myths about its requirements. One of the more widely spread myths claims that businesses will face financial ruin if they are required to provide physical access to their facilities. Since the adoption of the ADA, there have been no reported business failures because of financial hardships incurred in meeting the standards for accessibility. Furthermore, providing access to all customers usually creates more business for them.

Secondly, another myth related to costs says that all buildings, not just those under new construction or major renovation, must be made accessible. In actuality, renovations to existing buildings are not required if these modifications are not readily achievable or represent an undue hardship on the company.

Another myth upheld through the media is that making public buildings accessible is a waste of money because very few persons with disabilities ever use them. None of the provisions of the ADA are connected to a requirement for minimum usage. As more buildings become accessible, larger numbers of people with disabilities will use them. Lack of access has prohibited people with disabilities from choosing what building they want to enter, or what services they want to receive. These access features also serve the entire community which includes the elderly, mothers with strollers, and even delivery persons.

The shape of the ADA's future will ultimately be determined by those who are affected by it most–persons with disabilities and their families. Implementation of the ADA will require creative, ongoing education and involvement in grassroots advocacy. When seventy percent of those who are directly affected by the ADA are reported to be unfamiliar with its purpose and provisions, there is much more work to do.

The disability community must continue to implement the ADA so that all Americans can benefit from these civil rights provisions. The Americans with Disabilities Act benefits everyone, not just those who have a disability. We all want our descendants to inherit better opportunities for success; that our economy will grow when we all work together; and that our nation truly remain a government that is of the people, by the people, and for *all* people.

For further reading about the ADA and related topics, the following books are recommended:

Bureau of National Affairs. *The Americans with Disabilities Act: A Practical and Legal Guide to Impact, Enforcement, and Compliance.* Washington, DC, 1990.

Shapiro, Joseph P. *No Pity: People with Disabilities Forging a New Civil Rights Movement.* New York: Times Books, 1993.

Nagler, Mark. *Perspectives on Disability.* Palo Alto: Health Markets Research, 1993.

Title I Technical Assistance Manual
Equal Employment Opportunity Commission
1801 L Street, NW
Washington, DC 20507
To order, write to the address above, or call:
(800) 669-3362 (voice)
(800) 800-3302 (TDD)

Titles II and III Technical Assistance Manuals
U.S. Department of Justice
Office on the Americans with Disabilities Act
Civil Rights Division
P.O. Box 66738
Washington, DC 20035
To order, write to the above address, or call:
(800) 514-0301 (voice)
(800) 514-0383 (TDD)

Transportation Information:
Department of Transportation
400 Seventh Street, SW
Washington, DC 20590
To order, write to the above address, or call:
(202) 366-1656 (voice)
(202) 366-4567 (TDD)

Becoming the Kingdom of God: Building Bridges Between Religion, Secular Society, and Persons with Disabilities: The Ministry of Harold Wilke

Compiled and Edited by Robert Pietsch, DMin

SUMMARY. This article profiles the life and work of Reverend Wilke. Career highlights and a selected list of writings are included. *[Article copies available from The Haworth Document Delivery Service: 1-800-342-9678. E-mail address: getinfo@haworth.com]*

KEYWORDS. Wilke-biographical, disability, religion and disability, advocacy, United Church of Christ

Harold Wilke has been building bridges all his life. Not bad for a man born without arms.

Yet Wilke embodies wholeness and healing. From early childhood, he learned to use his feet as hands. Wilke's eyes sparkle when recalling one of his earliest childhood memories:

> I was sitting on the floor in the bedroom trying to put on my shirt. My mother had placed the open shirt on a pillow, on the floor.

Robert Pietsch is Chairman of the Board, The Healing Community/*The Caring Congregation*.

[Haworth co-indexing entry note]: "Becoming the Kingdom of God: Building Bridges Between Religion, Secular Society, and Persons with Disabilities: The Ministry of Harold Wilke." Pietsch, Robert. Co-published simultaneously in *Journal of Religion in Disability & Rehabilitation* (The Haworth Press, Inc.) Vol. 2, No. 4, 1996, pp. 15-25; and: *A Look Back: The Birth of the Americans with Disabilities Act* (ed: Robert C. Anderson) The Haworth Press, Inc., 1996, pp. 15-25. Single or multiple copies of this article are available from The Haworth Document Delivery Service [1-800-342-9678, 9:00 a.m. - 5:00 p.m. (EST). E-mail address: getinfo@haworth.com].

I tried to get it over my head and shoulders, then down over my side. It was difficult! My mother stood there and watched me.

She saw my frustrated attempts, twisting on the pillow. But she lifted not one finger to help me.

Her friend stood alongside: "Ida, why don't you help that child?"

Mother said, "I *am* helping him."

Wilke learned early that it is our vulnerability which makes us strong. Now in his eighties, it is time to survey the ministry of this man who has been at the forefront of the disability movement for over half a century.

EARLY YEARS

Wilke began his seminary training just before the onslaught of World War II. With a travel-study award, he ventured to Union Seminary in New York; Eden in St. Louis; and the University of Chicago. Reinhold Niebuhr and Paul Tillich were his primary thesis advisors. Extracurricular activity at Union included Jewish refugee support services. He also participated in the publication process of Niebuhr's *Christianity and Crisis.*

A student publication carries this paragraph by Wilke:

Two months before graduation ceremonies, with a traveling-study award tucked in my pocket, I sought advice. Niebuhr's was blunt: "No one these days can afford the luxury of further graduate study. Go to work—chaplaincy or pastorate." Professor Tillich's was more pastoral: "Ach, Harold, it is too late; the war will come soon." I should have been more prescient: my first month at Union coincided with a young German graduate student named Dietrich Bonhoeffer.

Ordination was an event in which student became teacher. Clergy and laity alike discouraged Wilke to consider pastoral ministry. "How will you be able to baptize? Conduct the Eucharist?" Wilke, not to be deterred, demonstrated that by touching his lips from baptismal font to the person's forehead, the sacrament could be fulfilled. Years later, Nicole Fischer (lay president, Swiss Reformed Church) would comment: "Whenever we experience the Eucharist, we experience total participation . . . Christ himself called *all of us* to participate."

Orthodox Bishops asserted that priests must be able to make the sign of the cross:

"We cannot ordain a young man with a disability."

"But suppose a seminary student was wounded in war?"

"I think we could ordain him."

"What's the difference?"

(And a long silence usually followed.)

FIRST CAREER: A UNIVERSITY TOWN PASTORATE

Wilke began his ministry at The Chapel University Church in Columbia, Missouri. The parish served faculty and students of the University of Columbia College. The first woman to be ordained from his religious tradition (Evangelical and Reformed, now United Church of Christ) was one of his students. Wilke preached the ordination sermon.

Guest preachers at the Chapel read like a Who's Who: seminary presidents McGiffert of Chicago; Beavan of Rochester; Schroeder of Eden; and the vice presidential candidate teamed with Norman Thomas (Roosevelt won that election). President Albert W. Palmer of Chicago Theological School returned with a story: "Wilke drove me to several historic sites in Missouri, but never laid a hand on the steering wheel!"

During his tenure at The Chapel, Wilke was elected secretary of the denomination's social action group, headed by Professor J.F. Arndt of Eden. In that capacity, Wilke edited and assembled the first issues of *SOCIAL ACTION*, the United Church of Christ's premiere publication for many years.

SECOND CAREER: THE WAR-TIME CHAPLAINCY

World War II brought change for everyone. Wilke was by now married to his wife Margaret ("Peg"). The two of them left their respective responsibilities—she as director of the Family Service Society and he at The Chapel, moving to new work in Boston. Harold entered Clinical Pastoral Training at Massachusetts General Hospital; Peg assumed duties with the American Red Cross. Both were volunteers with the Boston YMCA and hosted soldiers and sailors preparing to ship out to war.

Four years of hospital chaplaincy for the Army followed, based in Boston and later in Philadelphia. In his spare time, Wilke finished his Master of Sacred Theology degree from Harvard University and Andover Newton Seminary.

Wilke's ministry to wounded soldiers—and the congregations to which these men and women returned—is noted briefly by Seward Hiltner in a foreword to Wilke's book, *Greet the Man*. Hiltner writes:

> Attitudes toward persons with disabilities are set forth here by a man whose insights come not only from his creative imagination, his religious ministry to persons with health concerns, and his experience as a parish minister; but also from long study of his own feelings and responses as a person we ordinarily call "handicapped" or "disabled." Although he has no arms, he has nevertheless developed deft ways of performing nearly all the activities which the person with two arms can perform.

The book's title reflects Wilke's oft-repeated injunction: "Greet the person—not the disability."

Moving to Kansas at war's end, Wilke served as chaplain at the Veteran's Administration Hospital in Topeka under General William C. Menninger, M.D. Wilke joined the faculty of the School of Psychiatry under Dr. Karl Menninger, M.D. Wilke went on staff as thousands of veterans were being reassimilated into society during and subsequent to the war. This era saw the beginning of medical rehabilitation as a force in American health care.

Menninger comments in the foreword for Wilke's third book, *Creating the Caring Congregation:*

> On the strength of Dr. Wilke's book sent me by Seward Hiltner, I invited him to lecture at the new veterans' hospital.

However lucid and cogent Wilke's writing, his presence makes it all sharper.

Through my door came this young man who introduced himself as Harold Wilke. I rose to greet him.

"I can't shake hands with you," he said. "I never had hands."

As he spoke, his face, smile, and friendly attitude conveyed more than any handshake could have done.

He brought forth a notebook from his side coat pocket, a pen for writing and acted in every way like a man who had no disability. "This is true," he said. "I was expected by my parents to do everything my brothers did, and I learned alternative ways—toes instead of fingers."

I was developing a concept later called "Weller than Well," and somehow I saw this reflected in Harold Wilke. Perhaps the physical disability that people see, in spite of his independence, enables him to understand people who must make special efforts to keep up. I invited him to join our staff as chaplain. Working with patients, his situation afforded an understanding of feelings they might not convey to the average visitor or doctor. Perhaps he could help all of us realize how disability can be overcome.

This he certainly did. Patients loved him; so did the nurses and doctors. He inspired hope and renewed efforts in hundreds of people. He influenced me, too: he made me ashamed of lamenting apparent lacks, incapacities and difficulties.

At the School of Psychiatry, Wilke penned "Maximizing Your Unconscious Support Systems." Reading Freud, he realized a striking corollary to the religious assurance of God's ultimate love: *The eternal God is thy refuge, and underneath are the everlasting arms* (Deuteronomy 33:27). Freud asserted the importance of constant early support, beginning in the womb. In Wilke's eyes, a sea of support is all around us from our very beginning, much of it unconscious.

THIRD CAREER: A SUBURBAN PASTORATE

Desiring local parish experience, Wilke moved to the suburban St. Paul Church (United Church of Christ), Crystal Lake, Illinois.

He led the church through major renovation, tripled its membership, and studied one day a week at the University of Chicago
toward his Ph.D. Much of Wilke's thesis became the book *Strengthened With Might* in the Augsburg Pastoral Aids Series, edited by
Russell L. Dicks. In his foreword, Dr. Dicks writes:

> We, who know Wilke professionally, think of him as a col-
> league, a person of wide experience, one with whom to ex-
> change ideas, carry on discussions and arguments. His congre-
> gants in a Midwest suburban town think of him as their pastor,
> not as an armless minister. [To all his parishioners], Wilke is
> an arresting personality, whose sermons and conversation are a
> challenge to them.

During this pastorate, he was elected a voting delegate to the
General Synod (United Church of Christ), first in a series of thirteen
General Synods. He also served on the Executive Council and the
"Toward the Year 2000" commission, setting the UCC agenda for
this decade.

FOURTH CAREER: NATIONAL LEADERSHIP
IN THE DENOMINATION

Wilke's proposal for a national "Commission on Religion and
Health" was adopted by the General Synod, UCC (St. Louis ses-
sion). It included other ministerial concerns: military chaplains,
continuing education of clergy, and seminary relationships. This
body was later renamed the Council for Church and Ministry (now
the Office for Church Life and Leadership). He was elected its first
executive in 1955 and moved to the national headquarters in New
York, where he served for twenty years.

Women in ministry increased in numbers. The Council set up
procedures to help women find pulpits and to overcome gender
discrimination in all aspects of church life. Guidelines and standards for ministry were adopted over the years by the two hundred
associations of the church nationwide.

Hospital and military chaplaincy remained close to his heart.
Wilke strengthened his denomination's relationship to its four
hundred chaplains through endorsement and local connections.

Overseas, military chaplains received continuing education annually at Berchtesgaden in the Alps. This responsibility occasioned considerable worldwide visitation by Wilke, often under military auspices.

Wilke comments: "The Army felt it necessary to assign a military rank to civilian consultants. I was usually given Major General status, so my staff car flew a two-star flag." Within the United States he preached at West Point, the Air Force Academy in Colorado Springs and often lectured on pastoral care at the Army Chaplains School. He later dedicated the Arlington National Cemetery Monument to chaplains killed in action.

Wilke's organization, *The Healing Community*, is a founding member of the Commission on Ministry in Specialized Settings. COMISS grew out of the institutional ministries of that period, and now lists thousands of chaplains and pastoral counselors as members.

A "Committee on Church and Disability," another Wilke creation, arose from his long-term commitment to justice for marginalized persons, as with women in ministry and black ministers. Marginalized clergy persons often have great difficulty securing a place to preach and serve. In response, Wilke and others initiated a churchwide support system for finding jobs. The nation's first "Access Sabbath Sunday" date was also set in 1976, making the cause an annual part of the national religious year calendar.

Grants for clinical pastoral education (CPE) and establishing CPE as a component in seminary training were high priority. Innovative methods were developed nationwide to honor pastoral ministries in congregations and for specialized ministries.

Wilke participated in demonstrations and marches, especially for Martin Luther King. Wilke's "arrest record" is from such demonstrations: at an anti-Apartheid peaceful demonstration, his companions in the police paddy wagon included Dr. William Sloane Coffin, then senior pastor of Riverside Church in New York. A previous arrest occurred at an anti-Nazi demonstration in New York City during seminary days.

FIFTH CAREER: BUILDING BRIDGES BETWEEN CONGREGATIONS AND THE WIDER COMMUNITY

The heart and direction of Wilke's ministry rests in the community. His abiding goal has been to raise the awareness of *institutions*, particularly in secular and rehabilitation arenas, about the spiritual dimensions of healing. *The Healing Community* was founded to aid congregations in their ministries at the local level. Religious communities are usually responsive, but frequently uncertain, about how to reach out to those who are alienated. These include persons experiencing mental retardation, mental illness, physical disability, the frail elderly, and others.

Twenty units were created across the country, many now under different names. During this period, Wilke wrote *Creating the Caring Congregation* (Abingdon, 1980) and *The Open Congregation* (1984). Interfaith seminars created by forty local groups over two decades have provided a major outreach for the accessibility cause nationwide.

Wilke's teaching in theological seminaries on pastoral care and counseling expanded under his new work with *The Healing Community* and its signal publication, *The Caring Congregation*. Over the years, Wilke addressed or lectured at many mainline seminaries across the United States and abroad.

SELECTED CAREER HIGHLIGHTS AND POINTS OF INTEREST

- On July 26, 1990, Wilke delivered the invocation at the signing of the landmark Americans with Disabilities Act. This is believed to be the first time that a prayer was offered at the presidential signing of major legislation. Wilke then accepted (with his left foot) the pen from President George Bush on the south lawn of the White House.
- Founding board member of the National Organization on Disability, Washington, DC.
- 1993 lecture in Rome before the Pope, Vatican leaders and ten thousand delegates from ninety-nine countries. (Editorial note: See the *Journal of Religion in Disability & Rehabilitation* Volume 1, Number 3 for the text of the Holy Father's address and other keynote sessions.)
- Address to the United Nations entitled "The Whole Family of God," which opened The 1980 Year on Disability.

- Served as officer and board member of The Independent Sector (the premiere organization on voluntarism in American Society) and twenty years for the National Health Council. For that organization he received the final presentation of the Carpenter Distinguished Service Award, which was then renamed the Harold Wilke Distinguished Service Award.
- Presented the Coulter Lecture at the joint meeting of the American Academy of Physical Medicine and the American Congress on Rehabilitation Medicine. Over one thousand physician-surgeons and clinical rehabilitationists attended the 1980 national meeting.
- Preached in over a thousand local congregations, from the Bronx (NY) to Orange County (CA). Countless pulpits abroad include Westminster Abbey and others from Hiroshima to Johannesburg.
- Helped create the "Shalom Shabbat" service, widely used in synagogues and temples.
- Advocacy for accessibility and inclusivity within Anglican, Free Churches and Church of Scotland within the U.K. led ultimately to the creation of CHAD (Church Advocacy on Disability) in England, Wales, Northern Ireland and Scotland. A London-based group within the Lord Major's Office, chaired by Lady Mary Hoare, the Lady Mayoress, invited Wilke annually to help in the thalidomide crisis.
- Three chief executives of the National Easter Seal Society, over the course of twenty years, refer to "the profound influence of Harold Wilke on the National Board." One noted: "You forced us to move from a 'service agency' to a 'Service *and* Advocacy Agency!'"
- Honors and awards too numerous to list.

Around the edges of these careers he has or still serves in a dozen other ways: teaching at Union Seminary and other graduate schools; Chairing the General Commission on Chaplains and Armed Forces Personnel; and serving on a dozen national and international boards of directors.

In fifty-five countries around the world, he has lectured or preached to congregations and voluntary groups. He ministered half a year in Germany (focusing on congregational and community responsibility in the thalidomide disaster); was consultant to the World Council of Churches; Protestant Observer at Vatican II; and active in the World Council of Churches. Wilke participates in the regular agenda of these groups—theology, education, social justice and peace, but always adds the dimension of accessibility and inclusion.

All of this career is supported financially by the groups for which he speaks. First support came from the Lilly Endowment which became, with matching dollars, a multimillion dollar grant. Additional support comes from writing fees and speaking honoraria. In recent years, honoraria and fees have gone into *The Healing Community* budget.

His wife Peg has for many years worked as a psychotherapist. Son William is a nuclear physicist; Christopher is a United Church of Christ minister in Long Beach, California; Mark is a designer-builder in Boston; John writes for *The Wall Street Journal*; and David is an environmental education officer for youth in the greater New York area.

Wilke adds a personal memo on the collecting, collating and editing of this document:

> It has been a joy—reliving rich memories of such varied professional activities to bring these reflections up to date. The first draft was done twenty years ago when I moved from Church and Ministry Committee [United Church of Christ] to The Healing Community/*The Caring Congregation*, Inc. The document therefore includes the insight, memories and data-checks of all my staff and colleagues.
>
> Taking that dust-covered document from the Archives, I continue to draw lessons from these memories (both painful and joyous) for the years ahead. This is another grace of the aging process. I thank God for the memories!

POSTSCRIPT BY DR. PIETSCH

Wilke's concern for disability arises in part from his personal situation: without arms, his toes do the work of fingers. With that "black glove"—a versatile tabi sock on his left foot—he is truly a "southpaw." (The tabi sock, of Japanese origin, fits around toes to provide dexterity.) He is completely independent in activities of daily living, flying alone to his various commitments. Such independence goes right along even with advancing years. In fact, the vigorous body activity involved in dressing, for example, may be a factor in continuing good health.

Wilke proclaims that it is not really his toes, but *imagination*, that makes independence possible. When friends of the paralyzed man could not take him in the door to see Jesus (Mark 2:1-12), they opened a hole in the roof. The imagination that seeks alternative solutions is essential for every person.

Wilke reiterates that the words we use are so important. Person-first language is best. For example, "person with a disability" is much more gracious than "crippled" or even "disabled person." As Wilke is fond of saying, "greet the person—not the disability."

"This too is Scriptural," says Wilke. "In the Christian tradition, Jesus responded to the blind man (St. John 9) in three ways: first, saying that the alleged cause (sin) was neither accurate nor relevant; second, that even in his situation he still could glorify God; and third, that something needed to be done about it."

So let it be with all of us: in our problems and difficulties still to glorify God, and *do* something about it.

SELECTED BOOKS BY HAROLD WILKE

Greet the Man. Philadelphia: Pilgrim Press, 1945.

Strengthened with Might. Philadelphia: Westminster, 1952.

Creating the Caring Congregation. Nashville: Abingdon, 1980.

The Open Congregation. Nashville: Abingdon, 1980.

Re-Imaging the Role of Clinical Training for Hospital Chaplaincy and Pastoral Care: Moving Beyond Institutional Walls to the Community

William C. Gaventa, MDiv

SUMMARY. The author envisions the emerging community roles of chaplains and pastoral caregivers in the ever-changing health care system of the United States. Particular attention is given to ministry with persons who have disabilities. *[Article copies available from The Haworth Document Delivery Service: 1-800-342-9678. E-mail address: getinfo@haworth.com]*

KEYWORDS. Chaplaincy, disability, religion and disability, community health, clinical pastoral education (CPE), pastoral care

INTRODUCTION

Chaplains and pastoral caregivers everywhere now feel the growing impact of community-focused health care initiatives. From my own experience, three vignettes frame this exploration of its implications for clinical pastoral training.

The Reverend William C. Gaventa is Coordinator, Community and Congregational Supports, University Affiliated Program of New Jersey (University of Medicine and Dentistry of New Jersey). He also serves as Executive Secretary, Religion Division, American Association on Mental Retardation.

[Haworth co-indexing entry note]: "Re-Imaging the Role of Clinical Training for Hospital Chaplaincy and Pastoral Care: Moving Beyond Institutional Walls to the Community." Gaventa, William C. Co-published simultaneously in *Journal of Religion in Disability & Rehabilitation* (The Haworth Press, Inc.) Vol. 2, No. 4, 1996, pp. 27-41; and: *A Look Back: The Birth of the Americans with Disabilities Act* (ed: Robert C. Anderson) The Haworth Press, Inc., 1996, pp. 27-41. Single or multiple copies of this article are available from The Haworth Document Delivery Service [1-800-342-9678, 9:00 a.m. - 5:00 p.m. (EST). E-mail address: getinfo@haworth.com].

Vignette One
Taken from my role as a chaplain and coordinator of religious services for a state developmental center in Rochester, New York

I remember talking to a local pastor whose congregation was located close to the new group home opened by our facility. He noted that during the previous week, he'd been at the mall where "I saw some of your people." The residents had also visited his congregation. The obvious question was "Whose flock do they belong to?" It was my hope that this pastor's congregation would come to experience and envision these people as "theirs," members of their body of faith. That, in fact, happened.

Vignette Two
From an experience as coordinator for family support

In Georgia, my work focused on developing new models of respite care for families. These efforts included tapping the enormous power of congregations to be "respite providers"–places of rest and sabbath for parents of children with disabilities.

I remember talking to a mother who shared with me about her frustrating experience with a local pastoral counselor. She'd talked with him about the difficulties of coping with her child who had a disability. "He wanted to focus on my relationship with my mother. I just needed a break." And so she terminated that relationship. She then directed her energies toward including her child in recreational programs for "typical" kids. As a by-product, she was then able to have a break from the constant demands of caregiving.

Vignette Three
Presenting at conferences for "secular" providers of services for people with disabilities

I am often intrigued by the way that increasing dialogue (among disability professionals) about the need to build community support and inclusion for persons with disabilities suddenly slows when you start talking about working with churches, synagogues, and temples. There are many reasons for that discomfort, not the least of which is a professional uncertainty with how to relate to the very complex world of faith communities. There is also a personal and professional uncertainty about whether or not it is permissible to bring spirituality and faith into the public domain. With health care shifting to the community, perhaps the faith community (as repository of faith and belonging) is a resource whose time has come.

THE CHALLENGE

One cannot talk about "natural" or "community" supports without acknowledging that congregations are—or can be—a huge resource for millions of people. Thus (with both humor and seriousness), I have at times introduced myself as pastor of the "First Generic Community Service Provider."

Whose people are "they?" What does pastoral care or counseling with people with disabilities involve? Who does it?

The move toward accessible community supports and community inclusion is being driven by the disability movement. Health care reform is only an indirect influence, albeit a significant catalyst. Chaplains and pastoral caregivers in disability services, such as developmental or rehab centers, who have not been able to reshape their roles to include community services have in many cases been the first ones without a job as facilities deinstitutionalize. That often leaves agencies with policies that affirm religious freedom but no resources or personnel devoted to assisting people with disabilities to participate in faith communities.

In the 1970's and 80's, the prime vision among the disability community was *normalization* and the prime devil the *institution*. Chaplains who had envisioned and practiced their roles as pastors to an enclosed and isolated world sometimes became symbols of "institutionalization." I remember talking with a director of a newer facility who was determined that his center become more than the traditional developmental disability model. He said, "Three things define an institution: a chapel, a bowling alley, and a barber shop."

As community-based services picked up steam, chaplains and others in the religious community battled to keep their jobs. The issue was too often addressed as maintaining what *had been* rather than reframing and defining the crucial role and skills that chaplains can offer in a system increasingly focused on healing and therapeutic communities outside of institutional walls.[1] The challenge goes beyond envisioning oneself as a pastoral bridge-builder to the community from the enclosed world of the institution. Pastoral care offers not just the skill of relating to an individual and their family, but also that of helping them reconnect back to the community . . . and helping the community "welcome them back."

Pastoral care with persons with disabilities thus became more than just helping the person "accept" his disability and "adjust" to her situation. As the Americans with Disabilities Act clearly symbolizes (and which people with disabilities affirm), the pastoral task means dealing with the stigmatizing conditions placed on people with disabilities by an unaccepting or inaccessible community. All too often, persons with disabilities do not feel welcomed and included *even in a congregational setting*. Pastoral care providers in the disability community are thus gaining clarity about their social and ethical roles. Their efforts increasingly focus on advocacy, inclusion, wellness and prevention in addition to counseling and recovery. One might argue that distinctions between "pastoral" and "social" ministries no longer make much sense. Each now occurs in the context of the other.

RE-IMAGING THE ROLE AND IDENTITY OF CHAPLAIN

There are a number of words and images one can use to describe these changes for chaplains. One is a title now held by increasing numbers of chaplains as "Directors/Coordinators of Religious Services/Spiritual Care." The title is certainly more descriptive. Another image is that of *Bridger* between facility and community. The pastoral role of bridging involves a shift of vision: rather than view a chaplain as one who stands with both feet planted in the institution, the chaplain has one foot in the service system (whether institution or community agency) and one in the religious community.[2]

One can take another step and envision chaplains and pastoral caregivers as having three legs: one in the service system, one in the religious community (ies), and one in a professional community of other chaplains and pastoral caregivers who are facing similar challenges.[3] The challenge and dilemmas facing chaplains in disability settings has simply been a prophetic preview of those being faced by chaplains in all health care settings as acute care hospitals and other institutions of human service move to a community focus.[4]

One difference between chaplaincy in acute care settings and those in disability services is that many of the "consumers" in disability services have been cut off from, or never had, the experience of being part of a congregation or community. A chaplain, rather than supplementing the role of a "patient's" pastor, has the task of facilitating a relationship between an individual, perhaps his or her family, and a community clergy person and congregation. Thus another image could be "match-maker." More theologically, one image that has been important to me is based on a word play that chaplains can assist in the "re-membering" of people with disabilities: that is, helping them to become members of congregations and community.

A more striking image, based on the Biblical symbol of community as "body," is that of chaplain as an "orthopedic surgeon in the body of Christ." Like the surgeon who reconnects a part of the body that had been severed in an accident or trauma, the chaplain helps reattach a part of the body to the whole . . . for the sake of both. Another, taken from the pioneering work of job coaches in supported employment services for people with disabilities, is that of "congregational coach."[5] This image describes one who works with both people with disabilities and congregational members to help build a relationship that taps the gifts and skills of both . . . and then knows when to get out of the way.

PASTORAL SKILLS IN A COMMUNITY CONTEXT

Changing the role of pastoral care in a community context does not mean giving up traditional pastoral skills but rather adding new ones or, as one might argue, expanding and reclaiming old ones.[6] In my early pastoral work with persons with developmental disabilities and their families, there were four key roles of pastoral care which summarized what they taught me about my role as chaplain. As I reflect more about those experiences, they appear to summarize pastoral care in general.

1. *Presence:* Being there at crucial points in people's lives . . . or even non-crucial ones. From the person's perspective, *"You visited me . . . "* At the core of a chaplain's or pastor's identity should be the audacious claim that "I bring God to people." The grace in this audacious claim is that people more often remember whether or not you were *present* than anything you might have said—however brilliant or inane. The challenge is maintaining that presence rather than having the right answers or trying to fix the situation.

2. *Guiding (or counseling):* Being with a person as s/he seeks to find meaning to the questions and issues within their lives, especially within the context and tradition of one's particular faith. For people with disabilities and their families, this often means struggling with issues of God's will; the role of faith in healing; the attitudes of others; and the struggle to discover purpose and hope.

3. *Shepherding:* It is the Biblical word for effective advocacy. A shepherd is both *caregiver* (using the traditional image of a pastor caring for his or her flock) and *searcher* . . . finding the one out of 100 who is lost or fallen between the cracks of caregiving systems. The shepherd not only walks through the valley of the shadow of death, but also wields a rod and staff. The chaplain/pastor thus may help families cut through jungles of red tape, fight off enemies who abuse, and help clear a path. The shepherd also "sets a table in the midst of my enemies." One could claim that the words of Isaiah and Jesus to "prepare the way, make the paths straight, fill the valleys, lower the mountains, and straighten the crooked ways" was in fact the first sermon on accessibility and inclusion.

4. *Mobilizing a Care-Giving Community:* Here chaplains need to recover the traditional pastoral skills of facilitating caregiving within a congregation, helping members to find their own gifts through caring for each other. The Mennonite model of developing circles of support in congregations (see their booklet *Supportive Care in the Congregation*) is an excellent example of this potential.[7] The development of respite care ministries among the diverse faith communities exemplifies effective mobilization.[8] These community responses allow us to rediscover the understanding of congregations as "sanctuary" and place of hospitality to the stranger.[9]

Mobilizing a care-giving community is also a skill where chaplains can learn much from the "secular" work being done in the community with people with disabilities. Circles of support, supporting relationships, friendships and choice, person-centered planning, and community building through natural supports are prime examples of such care.[10]

THE NEW CHAPLAIN

As chaplains look outward, they must take the role of assisting people with disabilities to become full members of community and congregational life. Their roles change from being representatives of a particular religious tradition within an institution (e.g., Catholic chaplain, Protestant, Jewish, etc., even though they may have related to individuals from many backgrounds) to a unique new creation. Chaplains must become aware, able, and skilled in working both on a *broad, ecumenical or interfaith* perspective while at the same time having the capacity to help people relate to *specific* congregations. Interfaith also means being a representative, advocate, and teacher about the role of spirituality and faith in an interdisciplinary, "secular" health care system.

The requisite pastoral skill, then (added to the traditional skills of pastoral care with individuals and congregations) is to *think ecumenically and act parochially.*[11] In doing so, several specific skills become crucial. They include:

1. *Consultation:* Find out what and where the resources are. Talk *with* community clergy and laypersons early on; don't show up late in the game plan with an agenda of what they should do. Begin with the assumption that clergy and congregations have gifts and strengths to offer others. Help clergy see that the same care provided to and with "normal" people is the same as needed by people with disabilities.
2. *Collaboration* means building partnerships and relationships with clergy and congregations. The link must be extended between service providers, advocates, self-advocates, and the religious community. Meaningful, enduring collaboration means looking at ways congregations can work together to meet the needs of people with disabilities, such as sponsoring an Interfaith Volunteer Caregiving Program in their communi-

ty.[12] It may mean, as many chaplains have begun to do, helping to coordinate a regional interfaith coalition of people committed to inclusive ministries to share ideas and resources, enhance awareness, and collaborate in new services and programs such as respite care or other care-giving ministries.

3. *Competition:* This notion appears to go against collaboration, but one of the facts of church, synagogue, and temple life has to do with friendly and not-so-friendly competition. (Secular providers and services call it state of the art or "model" programs.) Competition means being able to say, when appropriate, "If the Baptist church is doing it, why can't the Methodists?" Helpful competition means being able to point out ways that inclusive ministries bring new members and strengthen congregational life. And it means realizing that many people with disabilities (and their families, who collectively number more than fifty million people nationwide) are in fact among the "unchurched." Many families have turned to secular associations or activities because they have not been invited, welcomed, or supported in their faith communities.

4. *Coaching* is by far the most important role for chaplains and others who have been involved in what has been perceived as "specialized ministries." Chaplains can help others who are gifted in ministering, but who do not believe they have the skills to minister with people who have been labeled as "different." Coaching shifts the role of chaplain from being the *primary* pastor to that of recruiter, trainer, matchmaker, guide and sustainer of others in their ministries. Chaplains can also teach others (professionals, family members, and people with disabilities) to perform these roles in their own congregations.

There are a number of skills that one can ascribe to a good coach. Space does not permit me to describe them in detail.[13] Outlined below are four skills in pastoral and congregational coaching.

1. *The Chaplain as Poet-Artist* helps congregations and individuals explore their values and dreams. The chaplain assists in articulating those dreams in words or symbols which capture understanding, imagination, commitment, and feeling. It means shattering the jargon of service systems, translating professional language into

words and symbols that people understand. For example, "deinstitutionalization" is more meaningfully termed *setting the captives free* or *bringing the exiles home.* "Integrating people with this or that disability" into congregations takes on new meaning when described as *hospitality to the stranger.*

Such language is at the heart of faith traditions and basic community care. Congregations and sanctuaries are *places of welcome, refuge, and worship* and help others to be re-membered into the body of the people of God. The poet asks:

- What are the core values and questions of this congregation and community?
- What are the core symbols or metaphors of a particular tradition?
- How do we embody and integrate them in life and practice?

2. *The Chaplain as Witness:* In many religious traditions, to "witness" is to share or tell one's own story of transforming experiences within a personal journey. Bearing witness means telling stories about the experiences in relationships with people with disabilities. These stories may be very personal and reflect key moments which have shaped your work. A witness recognizes that shared stories create bonds in ways which theories and ideologies cannot, stories which incarnate real people and feelings.

It is not easy for professionals in disability services to reach this depth, for professional languages and role images have often precluded that personal vulnerability. Being witness means recognizing that "professional" does not mean "value-free." Rather, *profess*-ional may mean value-clear, willing to profess what one believes and why. One is then able to tell the stories of how that commitment came to be. Professionals enrich the caring relationship when they share the ways that people with disabilities have enhanced their lives—just as professionals have served "them."

3. *The Chaplain as Guide* serves both people with disabilities and their families, helping them access and fit into particular congregational settings. The chaplain also guides people without disabilities, inviting them into relationships with people who have disabilities. For some, this journey feels like an entrance into a strange, foreign, or scary world. The chaplain-guide does not "fix" but invites: he or she

models with patience, welcomes all questions, and helps others find their own gifts and skills. A crucial role is learning how to reverse the questions that people may have about people with disabilities, so that a question about "them" becomes a question for everyone.[14] We must recognize that people with disabilities are in fact our guides into a land where we are all pushed to look at fundamental questions about faith, community, and humankind. Thus, the question may go beyond how "we" serve as spiritual guides to people with disabilities to a more profound reversal: "How do 'they' serve as 'our' guides?"

4. *The Chaplain as Celebrant:* The celebrant is a traditional religious role in worship and congregational life. In chaplaincy and pastoral care, *celebrant* also means helping people find ways to celebrate even when progress seems slow, to recognize the value of celebrations as a way of building community. Most of all, the chaplain-celebrant helps people discover the gifts and potential inherent in both people with disabilities (who are too often defined through their deficits) as well as the gifts in congregations or communities too often defined as uncaring. Celebration means a recovery of what John McKnight calls "capacity vision"[15] and what Parker Palmer describes as envisioning "abundance in community rather than scarcity."[16] It means finding ways to celebrate accomplishments, growth, new revelations, memberships, struggles, and rites of passage through ritual, party, and song.[17]

IMPLICATIONS FOR TRAINING

The community setting calls for a variety of skills to effect bridging and "congregational coaching." The implications run deep for training a host of professionals: chaplains, pastors, and others in human services and health care. These training needs are perhaps obvious, but let me list a few.

1. *New focus on helping students understand and access the community.* Training in pastoral care needs to focus on more than one-to-one pastoral relationships, as has been the tradition in clinical pastoral education and pastoral counseling. Emphasis must be given to skills in community building, collaboration, networking, and coaching others. So much of clinical pastoral education (CPE)

has focused on what people learn about pastoral care with individuals and families in acute care, crisis situations. This element of CPE training needs to be balanced with pastoral skills in ministries that sustain others over the long haul.

2. *Expand CPE training sites into community settings.* Training which has usually taken place with individuals in a hospital or institutional setting needs to move its location, so that at least part of the training occurs in a community context. Aspiring chaplains become bridge builders in service systems: they have one leg in the service system and one in the community. Students learn from experiences of integrating the two ministry arenas as they assist people with disabilities (and those without) in efforts to become a more caring, inclusive community.

3. *Chaplains must teach other health care professionals how to recognize and address their clients' spiritual concerns.* Clinical pastoral training which has traditionally focused on being able to identify and claim the role of pastoral care and spirituality in an interdisciplinary team needs to broaden. Chaplains can teach other health care professionals—in a variety of disciplines—how to integrate attention to their patients' spirituality into their professional practice. This can be done through skills in spiritual assessment and the inclusion of spirituality, faith and congregational supports in "treatment plans," "discharge planning," or newer models of planning known in developmental disability circles as "personal futures plans" or "person-centered planning." Chaplains can also train professionals in other disciplines to be "church coaches" to their own congregation or to the diverse faith communities to whom their clients relate.

Chaplains can also explore with other professionals the ways that their own professional practice and sense of calling impacts, and is impacted by, their own spirituality, faith, and values. Many people move into professional human services because of values learned in childhood in faith communities. Whatever the course of their faith journeys, most adults have not had training models which sanction the integration of spirituality into their professional lives. Chaplains thus become resources to many of these *profess*-ionals, not simply the one expected to deliver all spiritual care. While one might wish for ample funding of chaplaincy staff to deliver all those services, it will not happen; nor should it, if we are serious about stewardship of resources and, more importantly, the integration of spirituality into all avenues of care and support.

4. *Provide students with training which addresses not only inter-personal relationships but a keen awareness of community systems and organizations.* Traditional pastoral care education has included experience and skills in group dynamics through such arenas as interpersonal relationship groups, group therapy, and support groups. Again, this training needs to be supplemented and broadened by understandings of organizational and systems dynamics. Students must also become skilled at envisioning and shaping community building.

For example, IPR (interpersonal relations) groups in clinical pastoral education have focused on individual growth in a group context of consultation, confrontation, and support. Students are much better served when they are able to connect their group process to the role of groups and communities in sustaining the care and growth of persons (including pastors) over the long haul. Rather than "fixing weakness or limitations," we learn from people with disabilities that community building has to focus on gifts and strengths. We must teach students the value of sustaining one another when some limitations or "chronic" conditions cannot be fixed. Many limitations faced by people with disabilities are contextual (e.g., architecture and transportation) and social (e.g., attitudes, stereotypes, and lack of friendships). These social structures need changing or fixing as well.

5. *Stress the pastoral role of empowerment.* Training in pastoral care and chaplaincy needs to focus on the crucial skills of empowering others. Empowering means not only listening to people with disabilities and their families but also assisting them to try again to get involved in a faith community of their choice and tradition. It means recruiting, training, and guiding others—whether clergy, lay people, or other professionals—to develop their own capacities to minister to and with people with disabilities and their families. The irony is that too often clergy and congregations feel "disabled" in their ability to minister with people with disabilities.

Most importantly, empowerment means helping everyone see and find the ways that people with disabilities can in fact minister to we who are *TABs* ("temporarily able-bodied"), as Harold Wilke would say through the contributions they make to other individuals, congregations, and communities.

CONCLUSION

Community-based care has created a rapidly changing system of services and supports. This article has briefly explored the challenges, skills, and training issues for clinical education of chaplains and clergy in this context, with particular attention to the disability movement. I would like to make two points in conclusion.

The first is simply to reiterate a point that has been more implicit than explicit in this discussion. These challenges and training issues are not just for chaplains but also for community clergy, and, if learned, are skills which enhance pastoral care and leadership in whatever arena one ministers and serves.

Second, our debt to Harold Wilke's pioneering leadership is immense. In his career, Wilke first moved from chaplaincy in institutional and specialized settings to ministry within denominational structures. He then developed one of the first ministries whose explicit role was to build bridges from institutions to communities. *The Healing Community* models how bridges can be built between hospitals, agencies, advocates, and families to tap the healing potential of caring congregations. Much of his ministry was also within "secular systems." Wilke has long provided leadership through consultation, collaboration, and coaching which has called both professionals and political leaders to embrace the importance of spirituality and faith.[18]

That leadership has been evident in rehabilitation and advocacy networks; the United Nation's International Year of Persons with Disabilities in 1981; and is captured most poignantly in the blessing and signing of the Americans with Disabilities Act of 1990. Harold has been very clear that his primary identity is pastor and clergy, and thus has been able to call and guide people from many different faith groups.

Perhaps most evident to all who have been influenced by him, Harold Wilke's contribution has been to witness not only through his personal abilities but also his willingness to share his personal stories in a way that has inflamed hope. He has helped many people to celebrate the real and potential gifts of people too often dismissed simply as "disabled" or "handicapped." In that, he has simply been one of the first to help all of us in pastoral ministry to remember that our first task is to listen. We are then called to help others discover and respond to their understanding of God's *presence* in their lives—and God's call to use their gifts in ministry and service to others.

NOTES

1. See the *Georgia Site Visit Team Report* of the Public Issues Task Force, Congress on Ministries in Specialized Settings (COMISS), July 1992. This report outlined what happened when the State of Georgia eliminated chaplaincy positions *en masse* in psychiatric hospitals, state rehab centers, developmental centers, and some prisons. For a copy, write Bill Gaventa, 31 Alexander Street, Princeton, NJ 08540. (Include a self-addressed, stamped 10" × 13" envelope with $1.25 postage.)

2. See a "White Paper on the Role of Chaplains" developed by the Office of Mental Retardation and Developmental Disabilities in New York. Contact: The Reverend Jean Jenkins, 10-1 Selden Street, Rochester, NY 14605. See also excerpts in the Fall 1995 issue of the newsletter *Networks*, Post Office Box 685, Cocoa, FL 32923.

3. Gaventa, W. (1995). "Where Two Are Connected in the Presence of a Third: The Potential of Professional Pastoral Association(s), in *Journal of Supervision and Training in Ministry*, Volume 16, 1995.

4. For example, see "One Hospital's Changing Terrain" by Deacon Art Metallo in *Vision* (The Newsletter of the National Association of Catholic Chaplains), Volume 5, Number 1, January 1995. See also "Building Legs for a Combined Future" by The Reverend Joseph Driscoll, *Vision*, Volume 5, Number 5, May 1995.

5. Gaventa, William (1989). "Bring on the Church Coach," in *AAMR News and Notes*, Summer Issue.

6. Gaventa, William (1993). "Gift and Call: Recovering the Spiritual Foundations of Friendships," in *Friendships and Community Connections Between People With and Without Developmental Disabilities*, ed. Angela Novak Amado. Baltimore: Brookes Publishing Company, pp. 41-66.

See also McKnight, John (1995), "The Backwardness of Prophets," and "Christian Service in *The Careless Society: Community and Its Counterfeits* (Basic Books, 10 East 53rd Street, New York, NY 10022-5299.

7. Preheim-Bartel, Dean and Neufeld, A. *Supportive Care in the Congregation*. Cost: one to five copies available free of charge from Mennonite Mutual Aid–Advocacy and Educational Resources, Box 483, Goshen, IN 46527.

8. Van Dyken, Bill. "Respite Care in the Religious Community." *Exceptional Parent Magazine*, Volume 25, Number 7, July 1995, pp. 41-43.

Gaventa, William (1990). "Respite Care: The Opportunity for State-Church Partnership." *Exceptional Parent Magazine*, Volume 20, Number 4, June 1990, pp. 22-26.

9. Palmer, Parker (1983). *The Company of Strangers: Christians and Renewal of America's Public Life*. New York: Crossroads Publishing Company.

10. There is a vast new literature here, but see, for examples, the books from Communitas, 730 Main Street, Manchester, CT 06045 such as *The Whole Community Catalogue*, *Ways of Welcome*, *Capacity Works*, and the *Community Connections Resource Guide*.

See also the works by John McKnight and colleagues, such as *The Gift of Hospitality: Opening Doors of Community Life to People With Disabilities* and *Getting Connected* by Mary O'Connell; *Building Community Capacity From the Inside Out* by John Kretzmann and John McKnight from the Center for Urban Affairs and Policy Research, Northwestern University, 2040 Sheridan Road, Evanston, Illinois 60208-4100.

11. Gaventa, William. "Think Ecumenically, Act Parochially." Unpublished paper available from the author.

12. For program development materials, information on available start-up grants, and technical assistance contact: National Federation of Interfaith Volunteer Caregivers, Inc., Post Office Box 1939, Kingston, NY 12401.

13. For a more detailed description of these roles, see the paper mentioned earlier, "Think Ecumenically, Act Parochially" or "Gift and Call: Recovering Spiritual Foundations of Friendships," in *Friendships and Community Connections Between People With and Without Developmental Disabilities*, Ed. Angela Novak Amado. Baltimore: Brookes Publishing Company, 1993, pp. 41-66.

14. Gaventa, William (1986). "Religious Ministries and Services with Adults with Developmental Disabilities," in *The Right to Grow Up*, Ed. Jean Ann Summers. Baltimore: Brookes Publishing Company.

15. McKnight, John (1995). "Do No Harm" and "Regenerating Community," in *The Careless Society: Community and Its Counterfeits*.

16. Palmer, Parker (1992). *The Active Life: A Spirituality of Work, Creativity, and Caregiving*. New York: Harper and Row.

17. For example, the cassette tape, "Connections" by Tom Hunter. Available from The Song Growing Company, 1225 East Sunset Drive, Bellingham, WA 98226 produced in collaboration with the Beach Center on Families and Disability, University of Kansas. Or, Unpublished Paper and Presentation, "What's Our Song?," by William Gaventa, available from the author.

18. Editor's Note: To further explore the course of Wilke's career and its influence on the field of religion and disability, see the article included in this volume written by Robert Pietsch.

What the ADA Teaches Us About the Value of Civil Rights

Joseph P. Shapiro, BA, MS

SUMMARY. The author weaves both history and human drama in his illustration of our nation's most significant civil rights legislation since the sixties. This article tangibly portrays how a law affects the life of a human being–and its meaning for all Americans. *[Article copies available from The Haworth Document Delivery Service: 1-800-342-9678. E-mail address: getinfo@haworth.com]*

KEYWORDS. Disability, Americans with Disabilities Act, ADA, civil rights

Former Chicago firefighter Dennis Bell does not consider himself "disabled." Nor does he claim membership in the disability civil rights movement that won passage of the Americans with Disabilities Act (ADA). But the way Bell and thousands of others are using the ADA is a reminder of the original promise of all civil rights laws.

Bell sued under the ADA to be reinstated to the Chicago fire

Joseph P. Shapiro is a senior editor at *U.S. News and World Report* and author of *No Pity: People with Disabilities Forging a New Civil Rights Movement* (Times Books, 1993). Mr. Shapiro has written widely on social and policy issues. His work has appeared in the *Washington Post, The Progressive, The Disability Rag*, and many other publications.

[Haworth co-indexing entry note]: "What the ADA Teaches Us About the Value of Civil Rights." Shapiro, Joseph P. Co-published simultaneously in *Journal of Religion in Disability & Rehabilitation* (The Haworth Press, Inc.) Vol. 2, No. 4, 1996, pp. 43-46; and: *A Look Back: The Birth of the Americans with Disabilities Act* (ed: Robert C. Anderson) The Haworth Press, Inc., 1996, pp. 43-46. Single or multiple copies of this article are available from The Haworth Document Delivery Service [1-800-342-9678, 9:00 a.m. - 5:00 p.m. (EST). E-mail address: getinfo@haworth.com].

43

department. Fighting a fire in 1975, Bell fell fifteen feet through a collapsing stairwell and shattered his ankle. As time passed, he missed the close-knit bonds among his fellow Irish-American firemen from Chicago's South Side and longed to return to the firehouse. So to get off disability leave and go back to work, Bell, a Vietnam veteran, chose to undergo nearly thirty surgeries in a macho attempt to heal his injuries. Those operations failed and finally in 1991 the leg was amputated.

The new prothesis turned out to be a revelation. Bell's leg pains were gone, he walked without a limp, he could dance again with his wife and play golf with his buddies. The artificial leg, along with his discovery of the ADA, made Bell reject his own reflexive shame of disability. For seventeen years he had sought cures; he now sought accommodations. The passage of the ADA represented a similar two decade change of self-image in the disability movement: persons with disabilities came to reject the label of patient and demanded to be full participants in daily American life.

Like most Americans, Bell was unaware of this history, unaware that a civil rights movement was growing around disability. So when a friend in 1991 showed him an article about the ADA, Bell was unfamiliar with the law won by disability rights activists. The landmark legislation was designed to extend to Americans with disabilities the same protections against discrimination in the workplace, public accommodations and government services already guaranteed to racial, religious and ethnic minorities and to women.

Bell knows he can no longer be expected to climb one hundred foot ladders or drag hoses into burning buildings, but that part of firefighting is a young man's game, anyway. He can, as he argued in his lawsuit, take a different job–like investigating arson, training young recruits at the firefighter's academy, or working as a driver or dispatcher. "I have a prothesis. Okay, big deal," says Bell. "I walk and I'm doing fine."

Such use of the ADA–by people who do not consider themselves part of the disability civil rights movement–shows the power of the disability movement to change the way Americans consider civil rights. Today, civil rights have come to be seen as belonging to specific constituencies. Fairly or not, civil rights are equated with group rights. The disability movement, however, is a reminder that all Americans have a mutual investment in protecting civil rights. As people with disabilities point out, anyone can join the nation's population of 49 million persons with disabilities at any time, and as we live longer our odds of doing so increase.

As Bell sees it, he was insisting on simple fairness and common-sense, rather than waging a civil rights battle. But the ADA is also a reminder of the original promise of such rights movements: that people are to be seen as individuals–judged by the content of their character–not stereotyped on the basis of factors like race, gender or ethnicity. That is why the ADA forces an employer to look first at an applicants' talents and qualifications, and only then consider whether and how the disability can be accommodated. Bell knows that a man whose left leg has been amputated below the knee can still have skills and experience to offer the fire department.

The ADA was passed with talk of bringing down what one 1986 poll showed is a 66 percent unemployment rate among Americans with disabilities. Yet it is not the unemployed persons with disabilities who most use the law. Rather it is working Americans who get a disability, usually a minor one, later in life. Back problems, not spinal cord injuries, make up the largest category among workplace discrimination complaints. And of the first 25,000 complaints filed with the Equal Employment Opportunity Commission, 88 percent came from people already in a job.

After a three-year introduction period, federal agencies in 1993 stepped up enforcement of the new civil rights law. The range of disabilities and chronic illnesses covered by the ADA is displayed in the array of Justice Department suits and settlements. Owners of the Empire State Building agreed to make its observation decks accessible to wheelchair users; a state board of examiners gave a woman with a learning disability extra time to complete the licensed clinical social worker test; an Illinois city agreed to reinstate a custodian who had been fired after having a seizure; a drugstore chain changed its no pets policy to allow people into the store who used guide dogs; a Phoenix trade school agreed to provide a scholarship for the student it had turned down with a visual impairment; the nation's largest review courses for the bar and certified public accountants' exams agreed to provide interpreters for deaf students; and the city of Philadelphia instituted HIV treatment training to all of its emergency medical workers and firefighters after paramedics had refused to lift a man with AIDS onto a stretcher.

The EEOC pursued cases with a similar breadth. An Illinois security company was forced to pay the executive it fired because he had terminal cancer; pension funds and health programs were challenged that denied or limited payment of expenses for AIDS-related illnesses; a chemical manufacturer was sued for refusing to give flexible work hours to a man with bipolar disorder, or manic depression; and a Rhode Island state mental retardation facility was told to rehire a woman who was fired because she had a severe weight problem.

Most Americans, even those with disabilities, still do not know about the ADA, despite the fact that it is arguably the nation's most significant civil rights law since the 1964 Civil Rights Act. A 1994 poll by the National Organization on Disability found that only 40 percent of adults with disabilities have heard of the ADA. But based on its usage by those familiar with the law, the ADA can make the workplace and society more fair and generous for all.

For Dennis Bell, fairness came on October 15, 1994 when the city of Chicago settled his lawsuit and he began a new job: teaching safety to Chicago school kids. "It means so much to be back at work and be part of society," says Bell, "because people then forget about your disability."

ADA and the Religious Community: The Moral Case

Helen R. Betenbaugh, MDiv

SUMMARY. The religious community is technically exempt from the Americans with Disabilities Act of 1990. But is this an acceptable position for places of worship? This article examines the issues not in legal context but in terms of theology, moral teachings, experience and social justice. The author, a person with a disability, concludes with her own constructive theology. *[Article copies available from The Haworth Document Delivery Service: 1-800-342-9678. E-mail address: getinfo@haworth.com]*

KEYWORDS. Theology and disability, social justice, Americans with Disabilities Act, ADA, ADA and religion

In 1990, Congress passed the most significant civil rights legislation in 30 years: The Americans with Disabilities Act (ADA). Senator Ted Kennedy has referred to the law (PL 101~336) as the "Emancipation Proclamation for Persons with Disabilities." The ADA passed two years after its introduction and took effect on January 26, 1992. The law imposes far-reaching obligations on

Helen R. Betenbaugh is Director of Christian Education Ministries at Episcopal Church of the Transfiguration in Dallas, TX. She is Postulant for Holy Orders in the Episcopal Diocese of Dallas and candidate for Doctor of Ministry at Perkins School of Theology.

[Haworth co-indexing entry note]: "ADA and the Religious Community: The Moral Case." Betenbaugh, Helen R. Co-published simultaneously in *Journal of Religion in Disability & Rehabilitation* (The Haworth Press, Inc.) Vol. 2, No. 4, 1996, pp. 47-69; and: *A Look Back: The Birth of the Americans with Disabilities Act* (ed: Robert C. Anderson) The Haworth Press, Inc., 1996, pp. 47-69. Single or multiple copies of this article are available from The Haworth Document Delivery Service [1-800-342-9678, 9:00 a.m. - 5:00 p.m. (EST). E-mail address: getinfo@haworth.com].

private sector employers, public services and accommodations, transportation, and telecommunications.

Places of worship are technically exempt from compliance with this law. In fact, religious bodies lobbied for and received blanket exemption from the social standards of ADA (*New York Times*, Sept. 30, 1991). It seems almost frivolous to question whether or not the religious community has an obligation, with or without the strictures of the law, to meet its requirements. One could well argue that places of worship should have set the pace for secular society in the area of providing access.[1] The law's provisions should be a *minimum* standard for the religious community in its relationships with persons who have disabilities.

Sadly, places of worship often lag behind in all aspects of access. Physical barriers remain, as well as access through employment and basic congregational participation. Given that 49 million Americans[2] are estimated to have disabilities (1.4 million of those being wheelchair users), the societal proportion of *TABs* (temporarily-able-bodied)[3] to persons with disabilities is not borne out in places of worship. Persons with disabilities often can't get inside the sanctuaries to worship. The common argument is, "Why should our congregation build a ramp? We don't have any of *them* (persons with disabilities) who attend."

Briefly, ADA provides access to all public buildings (except entities which are exempt, including religious groups) for persons with disabilities under the following requirements:

- Public accommodations (restaurants, hotels, theaters, doctors' offices, pharmacies, retail stores, museums, libraries, parks, private schools, daycare centers) may not discriminate on the basis of disability.
- Reasonable changes in policies, practices and procedures must be made to avoid discrimination.
- Auxiliary aids and services must be provided to individuals with vision or hearing impairments or other individuals with disabilities so that they can have an equal opportunity to participate or benefit.
- Physical barriers in existing facilities must be removed if modification is readily achievable (i.e., easily accomplished and

able to be carried out without a great deal of difficulty or expense). If not, alternative methods of providing the services must be offered, if those methods are readily achievable. (Most modifications cost between $50 and $100.)

- All new construction must be accessible. Alterations to existing buildings must be accessible; including bathrooms, telephones, and drinking fountains.
- Entities which offer transportation generally must provide equivalent transportation service to individuals with disabilities.

Employment aspects of the law include a prohibition against discrimination on the basis of a disability and the mandate to make "reasonable accommodations" in facilities for all employees who have disabilities. This latter requirement affects only those religious entities with 25 or more employees, hardly a majority of the nation's congregations.

THE APPROACH

The primary focus of this paper advocates physical access to congregational property, facilities, and programming for those who wish to be a part of the worshiping community. Employment issues are not addressed. However, the issues presented have profound ramifications for employment opportunities. Additionally, barriers of attitude are frequently more excluding[4] than are physical barriers. While arguments for provision of physical access and employment opportunities stem from the same theological basis, the ramifications of both are simply too complex to address in this article. Lack of discussion of employment matters in no way signals that they are unimportant.

My approach in this paper will be both analytical and constructive. Scripture forms the basis for the discussion. The writings of St. Augustine and of Reinhold Niebuhr are employed to give evidence of the traditional/historical response of the religious community to ethical questions. Some of the most exciting new work, I believe, is offered by creation theologians, and so the third analysis will be on the work of Matthew Fox.

I also draw from the writing of Timothy Sedgwick, an author who represents my Episcopalian heritage. Sedgwick employs sacramental theology as foundational in ethical discussion. One could easily dialogue with a single theologian's work about the issue of accessibility, and in each case exceed the length of this entire paper. Only a portion of their arguments will be used here, but sufficient enough (I trust) to clarify their work as compelling and persuasive in the discussion of this particular ethical problem. My own constructive position will conclude the article.

Presuppositions

Before proceeding with arguments for the religious community's obligation to comply with ADA provisions, it is important to state forthrightly the presuppositions which I bring to my writing.

As a professional whose career in the ministry began at the age of 17 and as a seminary graduate in process for ordination to the priesthood of the Episcopal Church, the fact that I also happen to be a woman with a mobility disability looms large. As a professional in and member of Christian communities, I have experienced the gamut of reactions and responses by the religious community to my disability. These responses have ranged from judgment to condescension, apathy to pity, resistance to ignorance, compassion to confusion, from acceptance to outright rejection.

Second, I am persuaded that we need to set tradition aside where it speaks to us of the separation of body and spirit. Such dualism is counter-productive and even destructive both in theory and in practice. The Apostle Paul cites the problem of dualism frequently in his writings,[5] and this concept was given new impetus by Rene Descartes in the 17th century. The medical and psychological communities have been quicker to recognize the fallacy of such a split than has the theological community, though French feminists have done new and exciting work in the area of a theology of embodiment.

Though it is perceived as radical, theology of embodiment harmonizes with theologies of creation and of incarnation. James B. Nelson's book *Body Theology* (1992),[6] which addresses a number of contemporary issues from a self-consciously fully embodied viewpoint, joins the work of American feminist ethicist Carter Heyward. Heyward, Fox and others currently write "bodyself" and "bodyselves" to clarify that no separation exists between the person and the physical body. Ministry or evangelism (or anything else purporting to address my spirit) misses the mark if, at the same time, it excludes my physical being. Conversely, if my physical body cannot gain access to programs and people, then there is scarce chance that I will not feel rejected. In my faith tradition, Christianity is a religion of community–of relationships. The physical presence of a person in the midst of that community is therefore a given. Put another way, the body of believers is not complete if any of its members are not present when the body gathers.

Social Stigmas and Responses Which Exclude

The concept of marginalizing, of being ex-clusive (labeling persons who are different as set apart, as *other*) has its roots in prehistory. Here Mary Douglas' germinal work[7] (employing the disciplines of anthropology, political science, sociology, biblical studies and psychology) is crucial. Indeed, her analysis of the Levitical dietary laws demonstrates that the means of mobility were a major factor in deciding what was "clean" and what was "unclean." Social organization and the well-being of an individual are often linked to finding others of like identity and being. Thus *TAB*-society (the able-bodied) labels itself as normative and then, by definition, labels the disability community as *abnormal, different, Other.* When a group is kept at arms' length, they are not part of the community. Far worse, the community's obligation to them is seen not to exist.

Goffman's discussion of stigma raises many of the same issues. He asserts that persons with disabilities, being unable to conform to the standards that society calls normal, are then seen by that society as responsible for their own marginalization and oppression. Thus, there are both ex-clusion and moral judgments made against persons with disabilities because of those disabilities.

Intellectually and theologically, one might reject the force of such obvious wrongs out-of-hand. The following example eloquently decries that these judgments are both insidious and ubiquitous.

A woman who had been on a package tour sued the travel firm which organized her trip, because they had booked her into a hotel where a number of people with disabilities were also staying—which, she claimed, had spoilt her holiday. What is appalling about this incident is not the neurosis of the litigant—that sort of attitude is common enough . . . but the fact that she won her case. (Sutherland, p. 31)

THE BIBLICAL WITNESS

Ironically, the same Bible which pronounces Levitical laws excluding persons with a lame foot from approaching the altar also commands us to act in compassion and with radical inclusiveness toward persons with disabilities. It is further irony that, once persons have been marginalized, they become part of that community of widows, orphans, and strangers which the Bible repeatedly says must be treated with special concern. Indeed, the Bible testifies that God will take swift action on Judgment Day against those who oppress these persons (Mal. 3:5). Deuteronomy 14:29 commands that merciful treatment be given to the widow, the sojourner, and the fatherless. The stranger is among those to be given a tithe of the produce of the land in the third year (Deut. 26:12, 27:19). Scripture reiterates that God watches over the forlorn and needy (Psalm 146:9).

Israel as a nation is reminded throughout scripture that she was once a sojourner and seen by God in her oppression, and was delivered (references throughout Exodus and Deut., esp. Ex. 23:9). God's love for the sojourner is thus made explicit. Indeed, Leviticus 25:23 makes it clear that Israel lives by God's invitation, and so is always a sojourner in its relationship with YHWH. Taken in the full context of the Gospel, Matthew 7:12 (a passage known by the sobriquet "Golden Rule") decrees that the stranger is to be treated as God has treated his own people. Jesus himself made it clear that as acts of mercy are performed for oppressed persons, he himself is being cared for (Matt. 25). The claims of this story become even more compelling when one recognizes that, in Matthew's account, this is the last teaching Jesus did before his Passion begins.

The love commandment (Matt. 22:37-39; Mark 12:30-31; Luke

10:27) is self-sufficient in its powerful witness to the demands of the Christian life. Any person who her/himself experiences disability, or has a family member or close friend who does, wants the religious community to provide access for that person. In this way, s/he continues to live as a fully participating member of the community. Further, the love of God for oppressed persons has been demonstrated in the earlier citations. Loving with the love of God means loving the stranger. The Gospel of St. John 15:12 tells that Jesus required us to love one another as he loved us. Christ's compassion for the oppressed, especially those with disabilities, is evidenced throughout scripture.

Take, for example, the following construction of Jesus the carpenter. His concern for the marginalized, his passion for justice, and his care for persons who were ill or experiencing disability runs through the New Testament. Envision a modern-day scene with Jesus on his knees, pounding nails with his hammer, building ramps into inaccessible synagogues and congregations. He perhaps leads a team of volunteers in the manner of Habitat for Humanity. Jesus established a radically inclusive community in which those on the margins are loved by God. The Bible thus calls into question the objective and universal ethics of the natural law tradition (Cahill, p. 221). Rather than be expelled or repelled by natural selection, the person with a disability in a true community becomes the locus of the community's expression of justice and compassion, of *hesed*—hospitality and love.

In the Christian faith, Advent brings the radical message of God's love. The service leaflet at my congregation (for the First Sunday of Advent in Year B) describes a daily scripture theme as follows:

> There is a radical way to prepare and experience the joy of Christmas. It is to engage in the struggle for a world of justice and compassion—which is why Christ came. In so doing, we will find the kingdom of God in ourselves.[8]

Our lectionary readings for the Second Sunday of Advent include Baruch 5:1-9 and John the Baptizer's quote of Isaiah's prophecy (Luke 3). All of these speak of mountains being leveled, valleys filled up, crooked roads made straight, rough places made smooth. In other words, God desires to make his world accessible. Baruch says that this is done in order that Israel might walk safely in the glory of

God. Isaiah and Luke tell us that this is done to prepare a way for the Lord. In other words, accessibility is required for God's Incarnation and for God's people, so that "all flesh shall see the salvation of God" (Luke 3:6). Other New Testament material advocates this same requirement: "Make level paths for your feet, so that the lame may not be excluded, but rather healed" (Hebrews 12:13).

That same chapter of Hebrews (vv. 6-8) also addresses the ethical question at hand. Though it is decidedly unhelpful to name God as the cause of our hardships, the scripture claims that those who suffer do so because of their unique parent-child relationship with God. Persons who suffer are seen as legitimate children. One might construe that those who do not suffer can be seen as illegitimate.

Denying life to a person is tantamount to the sin of murder, as condemned in the Sixth Commandment. Luther believed that the worst thing that can happen to a human is not to hear the preaching of the Word (Carney, unpublished lecture, November 1992). One might also assert that happiness—the full personhood, the full humanity, and the enjoyments thereof—is a major goal of our life in community (a position which most ethicists hold). That which acts contrary to such maturation keeps a person from life.

The religious community puts the world's values ahead of the divine warrant when it fails to provide access and thereby disallows full life to the person with a disability (Carney, unpublished lecture, December 1992). Whatever denies, diminishes, or distorts the full humanity of a person is not only unredemptive, it is unethical and immoral.

AUGUSTINE AND ACCESSIBILITY

Carney's argument in "The Structure of Augustine's Ethic" illustrates that Augustine employed a double-matrix doctrine of love and truth (Carney, p. 28). If we take the command to love God, self and neighbor as fundamental to all discussions of love, then one statement alone makes a moral claim for access: "no one can love a thing of which he is wholly ignorant" (Carney, 30, quoting Augustine's *The Trinity*, 10.1.1). Keeping persons with disabilities away from congregational buildings keeps them from being known, and therefore from being loved. This is a direct violation of the "Love Commandment."

Augustine, says Carney, has a trinitarian ethic. Failure to honor one aspect of that ethic is tantamount to sin against God. For Augustine, the Son of God represents *Truth* and the Spirit represents *Love*. Some people acknowledge but do not embrace that persons with disabilities (whether those disabilities exist from birth or are the result of accident or injury) are created by God just as they were, and are loved by God.[9] Loving those whom God loves places an obligation upon one to love the person with a disability—a step which some people are afraid to take.

The historical Jesus "was seen to embody in His person a full and final revelation of the divine nature and activity" (Carney, p. 32). The care and loving concern which Jesus evidenced for persons with disabilities is evident throughout the Gospels. He interrupted other work to minister and heal; he expressed care for those who were even being turned away from him by zealous disciples. Luke relates that Christ told his followers to invite those with disabilities to their feasts. At the eschatological feast the rich and powerful, the "in" crowd, will be too consumed with their own activities to attend. The stigmatized, the marginalized, the outcast—yes, persons with disabilities—will gather around the table for the heavenly banquet (Luke 14).

The promise of the Holy Spirit in Augustine, says Carney, was not the promise of a power to evoke "new" truth, but the gift of insight into truth as old as creation (p. 32). The story of the origin of the twelve tribes of Israel has as its patriarch a man with a disability (Jacob), a limp from a displaced hip. For those who hold that disability is a result of God's direct action, this story is a wonderful refutation. Jacob is not only progenitor of the nation Israel, but he received his disability in a face-to-face encounter with God! The truth, as embodied in the historic Jesus, is that the poor and persons with disabilities are sought after and cared for in love. The Apostle Paul proclaims that in Christ, there are no divisions: no Jew nor Greek, no male nor female, no slave nor free person. We are all one in the eyes of God (Gal. 3:28). God sees people—not segregated as able bodied and others who have disabilities—he sees only people.

There is a principle in Augustine which has direct bearing not on the religious community, but the person with a disability. Such persons are often made to feel guilty, selfish, demanding, hostile, etc., for pressing demands about access to public facilities. The story of Lucretia was used as a statement against suicide, but more fundamentally, as an injunction against wrongfully accusing and judging a person and thereby punishing him or her under a false guilty verdict.[10] Just as Lucretia bore no guilt for her rape, so the person with a disability bears no guilt.[11] To assume second class status, guilt, or any other judgment is to submit to false accusations and pronouncements. The participation in false accusation and punishment is sin; the presence of disability does not indicate sin.

In *The City of God*, Augustine asserts that:

> A man who loves God is not wrong in loving himself . . . [and] he will wish his neighbour to be concerned for him, if he happens to need that concern. (Book 19, Section 13, p. 873)

Compassion for self is an entirely ethical position. It lies at the heart of the person's desire for access and of her/his actions toward that end. Augustine provides two rules: first, do no harm to anyone and secondly, to help everyone whenever possible. Both in his teleological principle of balancing good and evil and his lexically ordered deontology of obligation, Augustine provides ethical requirements for access.

Augustine also includes consideration of virtue in his theology. The example of Regulus[12] is relevant here. Just as he was judged to be virtuous (though not because he was not a Christian), so Augustine would see virtue in the members of Congress who voted for the passage of the ADA. Augustine would grant this virtue regardless of their religious affiliation or lack thereof, provided their motives were good. He would judge the religious community guilty of sin when it fails to provide access, failing to meet the requirements of its relationship with God. Conversely, Augustine would no doubt find special virtue in those congregations whose swift and enthusiastic compliance with ADA (better still, providing access before the law passed) was derived from their understanding of the nature of God and their relationship with God and neighbor.

REINHOLD NIEBUHR AND ACCESSIBILITY

Niebuhr's strong emphasis on the paradox of the rootedness/transcendence of human persons lends itself to the ethical question of access. He would, I believe, see disability as part of the rootedness which binds a person. At the same time, the person can conceive of something other than that state. The person can function in many ways as if the state did not exist, if access is provided so that s/he can function. This way of being is transcendence. Just as Niebuhr believed racism as a major crime (Carney, unpublished lecture, November 1992), so, I believe, would he regard failure to provide access. We are made as human persons, in the image of God. There is in each person the "stuff" of the Divine.

Denying that part of our humanity reflects the Creator is sin (Carney, unpublished lecture, November 1992). This reality has the same relevance to the person with a disability as did Augustine's use of the example of Lucretia (above). But this realization brings requirements for the religious community in its approach to persons with disabilities. That which is made in the image of God cannot be seen as Other or outcast. Faith (the opposite of sin) combined with love and justice provides the creativity needed to envision and then provide life in new ways for those not able to function within a TAB-based (the able-bodied) environment.

Niebuhr discusses various forms of pride which constitute sin or separation from God, self and others. The pride of *power* elevates the importance of self (for example, when the able-bodied (TAB) community sees its needs as more important than those of the disability community or the total community). This sin is the attitude which conveys, "I am better than others."

One of the most important aspects of Niebuhr's ethic is the normativity of mutual love, where the assumption of community among persons is basic. Here, the interests of others are to be served along with the interest of self (Carney, unpublished lecture, November 1992). This does not allow for exclusion. Furthermore, there is a dialectic here for Niebuhr: mutual love at times fails and needs to be temporarily replaced by sacrificial love, or agape.

Surely no person of faith would deny that Heaven will be equally open to all whom God welcomes there. If one understands that certain principles about life here will exist in eternity, Niebuhr says that their claim is equally important now, here in history. Thus, the same access that will be provided in the streets and mansions of Heaven must be provided here on earth. The return to the norm of mutual love should be easy once access is provided, for the person with a disability soon ceases to be *other*. His or her gifts become obvious to the entire community, and the question is then *How could we ever think of doing without Sue or Bob?* not "Do we have to include Sue or Bob?" The mutuality comes naturally.

Sin, says Niebuhr, is to deny rootedness and/or transcendence (Carney, 11-13-92). Thus, the religious community sins when it focuses on the rootedness of the person with a disability and ignores the dialectical claims of the person's transcendence. This same sin allows the religious community to delay or ignore claims for provision of access on the grounds that human persons can't right all wrongs and it will all come out okay in Heaven.

Real sacrifices must be made, particularly of funds and aesthetics in buildings which were constructed with total disregard of need for access. But there is no question that these sacrifices will create integrity of relationship with God. Failing to act sacrificially is to choose separation from God. Niebuhr's word:

> Mutual love is the harmony of life within terms of freedom . . . sacrificial love is harmony of the soul with God beyond the limitations of sinful and finite history. (Niebuhr, p. 78)

I argue that Niebuhr's sense of community and mutuality is so strong that the work done to provide access need not fall into the area of sacrifice. In other words, TABs (the able-bodied) who see the obligation of inclusiveness in their understanding of God would feel so impoverished by the absence of those with disabilities that they would seek, for their own good, to provide access. In a sense, this would be egoism, not altruism, coming out of a strong claim of mutuality.

Niebuhr's dialectic of love and justice has important applications here as well. Niebuhr took from Marx the argument that the principles of justice can be controlled by a select group so as to serve the interest of that group and not the interest of wider society. For example, just as black parents taught their children to "follow the rules" of segregation, so are persons with disabilities taught by many experiences (and reinforced by personal contacts again and again) that the world is made for TABs and their (the person with a disability) access problems should not become society's problems. The group in power, with no use of force but claiming the power of morality, can control the situation. Persons of color were discriminated against for years by a society which claimed its actions were just.

People follow norms in the name of morality. They also rail against those who refuse to follow those norms, such as activists who chain themselves to the gates of inaccessible buildings or who take part in human roadblocks along the routes of inaccessible buses. In this case, justice will definitely require some restructuring of society to produce the empowering of people with disabilities. Community is dependent on serving the interests of all. Nancy Eiesland notes that the civil rights struggles of African-Americans is similar to that of persons with disabilities:

> [The cry for justice] . . . calls into question the prevailing attitude that access and public services for people with disabilities were a matter of societal benevolence, asserting instead that people with disabilities have a civil right to access in societal institutions and public resources. It also began to dislodge the individualistic notions of disability. (Eiesland, p. 55)

> Access for people with disabilities is [not] a matter of benevolence and goodwill, rather . . . a prerequisite for equality and the foundation on which the [religious community] as model of justice must rest. (Eiesland, p. 67)

The African-American community has used the term *internalized racism* for a number of years. It is the situation described by Marx from the black perspective, i.e., the oppressed race supporting its supremacy by maintaining or participating in the set of attitudes, behaviors, social structures, and ideologies that undergird that dominance (Bivens, p. 15). The principle of *internalized ableism* is just as profound a problem for persons with disabilities.

Rules which address outcomes shift, Niebuhr argued. For example, the advent of birth control changed society's view of marriage and sex, but not one's obligation to one's spouse. Similarly, the advent of new surgical and medical procedures, new rehabilitation techniques and assistive aids have meant new rules for persons with disabilities. No longer is providing permanent care in a nursing home or rehab center acceptable for any but those experiencing the most severe disabilities. The new imperative is to provide access to as much of life as the person can and desires to undertake.

Niebuhr's arguments about the powerful inter-relationship of justice and love are such that he speaks to another access issue as well. TABs (the able-bodied) are inclined to plead ignorance to the needs of persons with disabilities. There is also the belief that if one is balancing needs and outcomes, the needs of persons with disabilities are secondary to many others. All of this changes when a TAB (or a relative or close friend of a TAB) experiences a disability. Access then becomes a major issue. The TAB is compelled to love the neighbor as himself and advocate for access with the same vigor (Niebuhr, pp. 246-247).

Niebuhr further says, "An immediately felt obligation toward obvious need may be prompted by the emotion of pity" (p. 248). While I know of no person with a disability who wants action based on pity, such awareness may still open eyes and minds. Love is the ultimate measure and motivator of justice.

> Equality as a pinnacle of the ideal of justice implicitly points toward love as the final norm of justice; for equal justice is the approximation of brotherhood under the conditions of sin. (Niebuhr, p. 254)

Empowering the unempowered was a primary goal for Niebuhr, the point of his ethical arguments on love and justice.

CREATION THEOLOGY AND ACCESS

Matthew Fox is a creation theologian, an area of thought which I find impossible to separate from creation spirituality. His synthesis of many issues surrounding community relationships and justice is powerful when applied to issues of access. Fox's style produces a gentle, right-brained argument that contrasts sharply with the more "rational" methodology of Augustine, Niebuhr, and others. As a former Roman Catholic cleric (now an Episcopalian in process for Holy Orders), his understanding is rooted in the sacraments. One of Fox's finest arguments rests in his use of the *Jacob's Ladder* vs. *Sarah's Circle* models of human community. Misreadings of the mystical tradition have resulted in a Western spirituality based on the hierarchical model (the *Jacob's Ladder* model). Instead of a quest for compassion, we have been given a quest for perfection. The model is one of moving up the ladder, toward contemplation of the Divine.

The story began with Jacob laying his head down on a stone for a pillow. His dream was progeny-, land-, and close-to-the-earth oriented. It was changed by male mystics to mean fleeing the earth to experience a distant, ascended God. The ladder puts compassion toward brothers and sisters at the bottom—away from God. At the top is contemplation of God. Perfection is upward—away from the body, the earth, matter, mother, and the sensual.

Feminist theologians reflect Hebrew understandings in their methodology. For example, *amongness* (not upness or exalted righteousness) is the dynamic the spiritual journey. There is the further notion that competition is not conducive to living in a Global Village. In circle dancing, we share ecstasies—not competitive combat. On the way up the ladder, one holds on tight to keep from falling. In *Sarah's Circle*, our hands are free to reach out to one other.

Worship as a visual image (just think about what body parts you see as you ascend the ladder behind someone!) summarizes the experiences of many in hierarchical worshiping communities. Worsh-up commands us to look up, shut up, and stay down. Worship in the circle allows us to look into one another's eyes, to sit in ways which invite all to participate as equals. The circle expands easily and fluidly to include new members.

Buckminster Fuller had wonderful words to say about circles. We live not on flat earth but a sphere. One doesn't put ladders up on spheres. Airplane pilots are among the few who use proper spacial vocabulary. They don't say they're flying up or down when they radio the tower; they are flying *in* or *out* of the circle. Physics has found no straight lines . . . only waves. A linear ladder, then, is an illusion (Fox, 1990, p. 50).

In the safe, sacred space of a circle we can be mystics. We can imbibe in the beauties, joys, and pleasures of living. Outside the circle we are prophetic: we go out to reshape society and history to better mirror the beauty we have received.

> In Sarah's Circle, God is not separate from the human dancing. God is found there, where neighbor suffers or is in need or celebrates. Justice is not separate from love nor is either separate from our love of God. God is in creation and in neighbor as brother or sister, or not at all. (Fox, 1990, p. 52)

Holiness, says Fox, is not a quest for perfection but cosmic hospitality. His view is consciously dialectical and specifically does away with the body/spirit dualism present in traditional religious writings. Where Augustine concluded, "the soul makes war with the body," Fox says (with Eckhart) that "the soul loves the body." His is a spirituality not of the powerful but the powerless. Rather than achieving purity by separating from the world, true spirituality is hospitality to all (Fox, 1983, pp. 316-319).

Fox's theology has a realized and not a future eschatology:

> Heaven is not so distant, nor so up. It is where people can learn to love as brothers and sisters, eye-to-eye, dancing Sarah's Circle and relieving one another's pain. It is wherever compassion is practiced. (Fox, 1990, p. 65)

Fox quotes Thomas Merton:

> The whole idea of compassion is based on a keen awareness of the interdependence of all living beings, which are part of one another and involved in one another. (Fox, 1990, frontispiece)

SACRAMENTAL THEOLOGY AND ACCESS

The classical definition of *sacrament* is an "outward and visible sign of an inner and spiritual grace." Sacramental theology teaches that through these holy rites (such as baptism and the Eucharist), God enters our bodies. Sedgwick's book opens with a quotation from Augustine:

> You are the Body of Christ; that is to say, in you and through
> you the method and work of the incarnation must go forward.
> You are to be taken, you are to be consecrated, broken and
> distributed, that you may become the means of grace and
> vehicles of the eternal charity. (Sedgwick, frontispiece)

Sedgwick's foundation for ethical discourse lies not in Scripture
(nor the nature and doctrine of God) but in worship. He sees *gift* as
the grace at the heart of creation and of the Eucharist.

> Our lives rest upon the initiative of God; our response is offer-
> ing of ourselves to God; our consequent experience of God's
> grace renews and impels us into the world to embrace and care
> for it . . . . Gift reflects the basic truth that John Calvin describes
> simply as the fact that 'we are not our own' . . . When the sense
> of gift is lost, the heart is distorted and with it the image of
> human life and creation. (Sedgwick, pp. 64-66)

Love is caring for life in its brokenness, but this is also a requirement of freedom. The person of faith is responsible to prevent the
continued misuse of power: "In the Christian vision we become
persons only as we are able to accept the other as gift, and in
response care for that person in trust and openness." Christian
ethics must be responsible and responsive to the claims of the
sacraments. Through them, we experience grace, gift, the community of faith, the inherent worth of each human person as a child of
God. In Christian tradition, baptismal liturgy asks the participant to
publicly affirm his or her intention to seek and serve Christ in all
persons.

> Justice demands responsibility for the social and political or-
> der in which we live . . . Love expresses unconditional care for
> each person. Since God loves all, justice demands that all
> people be treated equally. Certain minimal conditions for all
> people must be met to insure individual dignity. This would
> include, for example, food, clothing, shelter, and the opportu-
> nity to participate in the social and political order. Differences
> in opportunities and the distribution of goods could be accept-
> able only if all members of the society would thereby be
> advantaged. (Sedgwick, p. 91)

Surprisingly like the brief excerpt above from Augustine, feminist theologians value the body as a theological resource, while asking whether human physical differences ought to carry the theological significance they have come to bear (Ross, p. 186). Can one separate the sacramental signs of an inner and spiritual grace from the physical, the incarnational? Sacrament is by definition an outward manifestation of that which resides within the human heart. Excluding the sacramental expression of God present in the bodies of persons with disabilities (those seen as "abnormal") places human limitations on the sacraments, on God's grace. Reflection on the Incarnation in an imperfect body leads to new insights about God and the imperfections of us all. By experiencing the God who is in our bodies, we come to a deeper understanding of our creator—and ourselves.

A CONSTRUCTIVE MORAL POSITION: THE AMERICANS WITH DISABILITIES ACT AND THE RELIGIOUS COMMUNITY

My position is a synthesis of the above referenced views, and in other respects is a new approach. The Biblical witness for me is crucial and fundamental, not just for what it tells us about human beings, but more for what it tells us about God. It embraces and is fueled by the scriptural passages cited earlier. We all want to be included as we are; both the "Golden Rule" and the "Love Commandment" therefore challenge us to include others. Charity (love) shines when it is about empowerment, caring enough to give you the things I enjoy so that we can relate as equals. Love toward persons with disabilities, then, is not to be a handout. Love connects not from an up-down position, but through a hand reaching out—across the circle.

Any theology (moral theology included) is by definition God-talk. We are *all* made in the image of God. God's incarnation therefore includes body forms which are often regarded as imperfection: blindness, deafness, loss of speech, paraplegia and amputation, pain and disease, being female or Black, of short stature, etc. God is part of a person's pain and disability; such body states are sacramental expressions of God. God is a God of ease and dis-ease, of ability and dis-ability, of freedom and limitation, movement and stillness, of choices and imperatives, pleasure and pain; of joy and suffering, light and dark, of speech and silence, of running and being carried, giving and receiving help, of calm control and spasticity; of touching and being touched, hearing and quiet, of speech and silence.[13]

I am indebted to theologian Rita Nakashima Brock for the term "human flourishing."[14] The term decries a spirit/body split in one sense and in another conveys that just *being* is not enough. Human flourishing captures dreams for happiness, self-actualization, personhood, and full humanity. For the person of faith, flourishing is not possible without total access to the buildings, systems, and programs of the religious community.

While teleological, my argument defines benefits for communities of faith. When congregations better welcome and include all persons, the community is richer from their gifts and graces. Social stigma is a problem here; not all persons or congregations desire to include persons with disabilities in this way (cf. Sutherland example, p. 7, above).

Human flourishing speaks against the theology of virtuous suffering, which is apparent in society's approval of Lucretia's suicide (Augustine, op. cit.). It also forms at least a portion of the dialectic (referred to by Marx and Niebuhr) that moral complicity or acquiescence in one's own marginalization can likewise be traced to the idea of virtuous suffering. The prevalence of physical abuse against women has caused feminists to take a strong stand against such theology. It has unfortunately "encouraged persons with disabilities to acquiesce to social barriers as a sign of obedience to God and to internalize second-class status inside and outside the religious community" (Eiesland, p. 73).

In both scripture and the tradition, Christians have used *Body of Christ* as a metaphor for Christian community. Given this clear proclamation that the human body needs all of its members, it is indeed ironic that the Christian faith describes itself as experiencing the metaphorical equivalent of disability when any of its members are absent. The Body of Christ, the Church, does itself great harm when it cuts off or excludes persons with disabilities—its own members. The Apostle Paul often emphasizes the interdependence of the community of faith. Such "interdependence is not a possibility to be willed from a position of power, but a necessary condition for life . . . [It] is the fact of both justice and survival" (Eiesland, p. 103).

Religious traditions often carry a latent resistance to technology. Somehow these traditions still carry a subtle but profound distrust of things that are "of the world," no matter how they might help the people of God. Assistive technologies such as hearing loops, interpreters, or other adaptive equipment for persons with disabilities is receiving only modest introduction into worship settings.

CONCLUDING CONFESSIONAL

Before resting my arguments, I want to acknowledge the obligation of the person with a disability—persons such as myself. Whenever I respond as a "nice Christian woman" and ask nothing of the religious community for myself, I contribute to my own oppression. Niebuhr and Marx point out that a person, in good moral conscience, often participates in his or her own oppression in the name of morality. As African-American writers have used the term "internalized racism," so it is time that writers in the disability community name and speak of internalized ableism. God desires that I experience human flourishing, the full expression of the image of God within me.

Theologian John Deschner names our need: "I have sinned most often by not acknowledging myself as a friend of God." I have never experienced a lack of motivation to advocate on the behalf of others with disabilities; it is more difficult to advocate for myself. Lucretia took her life; I have often limited mine. The "virtue" of the death of even part of oneself is no virtue at all. One's obligation is tripartite: to God, neighbor, and self. The Golden Rule works for me too.

In short—look out world!

NOTES

1. The term "access" is used to include the following: full admission to congregational property and buildings; the presence of assistive devices and/or signed presentations for the deaf and hearing impaired; large print or Brailled materials

for the visually impaired; wheelchair accessible bathrooms; proper signage; and all devices, services, and materials which make full participation by a person with a disability possible. For simplicity, *wheelchair access* will serve as a metaphor for all access, including for those with emotional and/or developmental disabilities.

2. The estimated number of Americans with disabilities was recently revised to 49 million (up from 43 million). A printed envelope issued by the United States Postal Service, featuring a woman in a manual wheelchair and an urge to employ persons with disabilities, uses the estimate of 43 million people with disabilities as well.

Many people refuse to admit to disabilities because of the stigma attached to them. The term "disability" is used to include psychiatric disorders, AIDS, seizure disorders, respiratory conditions, diabetes and other metabolic disturbances, head trauma, sickle cell anemia, cardiac conditions, multiple sclerosis, muscular dystrophy and other neuro-muscular degenerative diseases, gastrointestinal disorders, allergies, the many forms of cancer, arthritis, chronic back pain, lupus, osteoporosis, glaucoma, retinitis, cataracts and numerous other visual impairments, in addition to the "standard" mobility and sensory disabilities (National Organization on Disability, p. 33).

3. In describing persons with disabilities, words like "normal," "non-disabled" or "non-handicapped" are problematic. First, they reinforce the concept of the other-ness of a person with a disability and reinforce continued marginalization. Second, they presuppose that those who appear "normal" have no disabilities. No one is unfettered from some sort of physical, emotional, or mental condition which keeps them from the full, free expression of their human personhood.

Preferred terminology is "person-first" language: *person with a disability* rather than *disabled person*, for example.

The term "temporarily-able-bodied" also includes recognition that the state of being able-bodied is not a permanent one, save for those who die young. In other words, if one lives long enough, everyone will encounter some sort of physical disability.

4. The disability community increasingly employs the word "disability" to refer to the physical difficulty of the person being discussed. The word "handicap" is used not in relation to people but to impediments: for example, the physical and attitudinal barriers which society places in the way of the person with a disability. Disability is a condition; a handicap is an obstacle (Maggio, p. 25).

5. The Apostle Paul does away with dualism of body and spirit, as reflected in his use of the words "body" and "flesh." His wholistic view often results in terms such as "spiritual body."

6. James B. Nelson is an ethicist at United Theological Seminary of the Twin Cities.

7. Mary Douglas, *Purity and Danger.* New York: Ark Paperbacks, 1988.

8. *Good News.* New Berlin, Wisconsin: Liturgical Publications, Inc., December 1, 1991, issue.

9. Viewing persons as *Other* (different, distanced, excluded) and stigma (cf. Douglas and Goffman) are crucial to dealing with the resistance of many persons to a positive approach to disability and to inclusion of persons with disabilities.

10. Lucretia, "a noble Roman matron of antiquity," was raped by the son of King Tarquin. She told her husband and her "kinsman Brutus," and asked them to take revenge. She, unable to endure the "horror of the foul indignity" and believing herself to be therefore no longer chaste, took her own life. This was celebrated in Augustine's day (City of God, 1.19).

11. Persons born with disabilities bear no complicity for the incidence of their disability. Persons whose disabilities are the result of their own illegal actions may bear responsibility: driving while under the influence of drugs or alcohol, diving into prohibited shallow waters, etc.

12. Marcus Regulus, Roman commander-in-chief, was a prisoner of the Carthaginians, with whom Rome was at war. He was sent to Rome by Carthage to plead their case in offering to free their Roman prisoners in exchange for Rome's release of Carthaginian captives. Regulus pledged to return to Carthage if he failed in his mission. He went to Rome, urging the Senate to reject the prisoner exchange proposal. He then returned to Carthage where he was tortured to death (Augustine, City of God, 1.15).

13. God's acceptance of all conditions (unconditional love) may be the Ultimate Reality of God and within me. Even the worst of my existence is of God, is in God, and God is in it. As some touch me, that touch is sacramental, and connects me and them and God. Even in my imperfection, I am also, paradoxically, part of God's infinite perfection. While I am Other, I am part of Holy Other. I can have peace with my own need to ask for help, for even Jesus said "I thirst" when he hung on the cross. I would never dare say that God was defined or limited by God's own "dis-abilities." Therefore the same is true for me, for I am made in the image of God. The person with a disability experiences the *mysterium tremendum et fascinans*, the fearful and painful side of God. Even where I am misunderstood and scapegoated, there too is identity with Christ.

14. *Journeys by Heart*. New York: Crossroad, 1991.

BIBLIOGRAPHY

Augustine. *City of God*. London: Penguin Books, 1984.

Bivens, Donna K. and Nancy D. Richardson. "Naming and Claiming Our Histories." *The Brown Papers*, 1:2. Boston: Women's Theological Center, November 1994.

Brock, Rita Nakashima. *Journeys by Heart*. New York: Crossroad, 1991.

Cahill, Lisa Sowle. "Feminism and Christian Ethics: Moral Theology," in Catherine Mowry LaCugna, ed., *Freeing Theology: The Essentials of Theology in Feminist Perspective*. San Francisco: Harper San Francisco, 1993.

Carney, Frederick S. "The Structure of Augustine's Ethic," in William S. Babcock, ed., *The Ethics of St. Augustine*. Atlanta: Scholars Press, 1991.

Douglas, Mary. *Purity and Danger*. New York: Ark Paperbacks, 1988.

van Dongen-Garrad, Jessie. *Invisible Barriers: Pastoral Care of Physically Disabled People.* London: SPCK, 1983.

Eiesland, Nancy. *The Disabled God: Toward a Liberatory Theology of Disability.* Nashville, Abingdon, 1994.

Fox, Matthew. *Original Blessing.* San Francisco: Harper San Francisco, 1983.

_____. *A Spirituality Named Compassion.* San Francisco: Harper San Francisco, 1990.

Goffman, Erving. *Stigma: Notes on the Management of Spoiled Identity.* New York: Simon & Schuster, 1986.

Govig, Stewart D. *Strong at the Broken Places: Persons With Disabilities and the Church.* Louisville: Westminster/John Knox Press. 1989.

Interpreter's Dictionary of the Bible. Nashville: Abingdon, 1962.

Maggio, Rosalie. *The Bias-Free Word Finder: A Dictionary of Nondiscriminatory Language.* Boston: Beacon Press, 1991.

Nelson, James B. *Body Theology.* Louisville: Westminster/John Knox, 1992.

Niebuhr, Reinhold. *The Nature and Destiny of Man.* New York: Charles Scribner's Sons, 1964.

Ross, Susan A. "God's Embodiment and Women: Sacraments," Catherine Mowry LaCugna, ed., *Freeing Theology: The Essentials of Theology in Feminist Perspective.* San Francisco: Harper San Francisco, 1993.

Sedgwick, Timothy F. *Sacramental Ethics: Paschal Identity and the Christian Life.* Philadelphia: Fortress Press, 1987.

Sutherland, Allan T. *Disabled We Stand.* Bloomington: Indiana University Press, 1984.

Thornburgh, Ginny, ed. *Loving Justice: The ADA and the Religious Community.* Washington, DC: National Organization on Disability, 1994.

_____. *That All May Worship.* Washington, D.C.: National Organization on Disability, 1992.

Vanier, Jean. *The Broken Body.* New York: Paulist Press, 1988.

Thoughts and Reflections:
Envisioning the Future
from the Guiding Principles of My Past

Harold H. Wilke, DD

SUMMARY. The author presents his hopes for the future, shaped by a lifetime of dedication to the field of religion and disability. *[Article copies available from The Haworth Document Delivery Service: 1-800-342-9678. E-mail address: getinfo@haworth.com]*

KEYWORDS. Disability, advocacy, religion and disability, Wilke

The hopes which follow in these pages come out of my own experience. Our society–humanity–has come a long way toward inclusion for persons with disabilities during my journey, these eighty-plus years. It has been a grand pilgrimage.

Allow me to share a few principles I learned along the way.

- *Believers, pave the way. Be visionary and inclusive.*

Nowhere is this image more cogent than the signing of the Americans with Disabilities Act on July 26, 1990. A visible image . . . did

---

The Reverend Harold H. Wilke is Director of *The Healing Community* in Claremont, CA. His career spans almost seven decades of ministry and advocacy.

[Haworth co-indexing entry note]: "Thoughts and Reflections: Envisioning the Future from the Guiding Principles of My Past." Wilke, Harold H. Co-published simultaneously in *Journal of Religion in Disability & Rehabilitation* (The Haworth Press, Inc.) Vol. 2, No. 4, 1996, pp. 71-79; and: *A Look Back: The Birth of the Americans with Disabilities Act* (ed: Robert C. Anderson) The Haworth Press, Inc., 1996, pp. 71-79. Single or multiple copies of this article are available from The Haworth Document Delivery Service [1-800-342-9678, 9:00 a.m. - 5:00 p.m. (EST). E-mail address: getinfo@haworth.com].

you catch it in the photo displayed in the front of this book? The President and Mrs. Bush on the platform, the Vice President and two longtime advocates of the legislation. Tireless efforts by Evan Kemp, Sandy Parrino and a sea of advocates who are bringing about the kingdom of God through social justice. Men and women, all races, all creeds.

For the first time ever, a blessing offered for a public presidential signing, a record host of onlookers.

Can you see it in the eyes of those gathered on the South Lawn?

The kingdom of God is ours to bring. Let us be found faithful and inclusive.

- *Assume the fullest independence, creativity and normality for persons with disabilities, right from the start.*

Years ago, the thalidomide disaster in Germany caused the malformations of countless newborn children. Thousands born without legs, without arms; many had heart and lung deficiencies. I was touched by the response of national and medical leaders. Dr. Ernest Marquardt insisted that his country do more than provide their children with prosthetic devices. No, he said: *we must see them as whole persons.* Consider their social needs; help them help themselves. Encourage them to be creative, innovative.

I could not help but recall my own childhood experiences. Having no arms myself, my *imagination* told me long ago that a coat is not only something that you can put on and button. It is also something that you can first button and then put on! So every morning, I pull my coat out of the closet and place it down on the bed beside me, face up. With my toes, I button the coat; next I flip it over face down, duck my head into it, and shake it down over my shoulders.

Given the chance, these children naturally went toward this approach: "Use everything you've got!"

- *There are enormous reservoirs of ability and strength inside every person.*

Sendai, Japan. Dr. Takahashi had scheduled me to address his pre-med students. My lecture concerned the professional hazard of knowing everything and trying to convey it to the patient. Since I write with my feet (I was born without arms), I invited them to join me.

Shoes doffed and pens in foot, they fought off untrained muscles and used their imaginations. Toes served as fingers.

"As soon as your seatmate can read your name, raise your hand."

Eighty-five percent of their hands soon shot up.

"Look what you've done! The same is true for your patients. Learn this—that your gifts, abilities, and strengths are tremendous in number."

Enormous reservoirs indeed!

- ***Professionals are laypersons and learners, alongside the persons with disabilities whom we serve.***

Several years ago the American Medical Association honored me with their "Layman of the Year" award. Accepting it, I quipped, "In *my* congregation, the medical doctors are the laymen."

Any professional who cannot (or will not) learn from her patients is missing a rich gift. We must never lose sight of our role as collaborators in the healing process: the living human document is our text. True enough, we bring specialized gifts and talents to the relationship. But if we are fortunate, the person will be helped—and our own lives enriched through the other person's gift of him or herself.

Can you still look into the eye of your client and see the emotions, the hopes, the dreams? They are yours as well.

- ***Help the persons whom you serve discover what nurtures them.***

When the late Drs. Karl and Will Menninger invited me to join their psychiatric rehabilitation staff, I came to have an appreciation for "oceanic feeling."

The concept is Freud's, and I immersed myself in it. Our basic rooting in the sense of nurture—being cared for—begins in the womb. For nine months, we float in a sea of amniotic fluid. Our every need is met, even though unexpressed. When we are born, the arrangement changes but the sense of nurture continues: when we're cold, a blanket is put around us. When hungry, we are taken to the breast. When in need of a touch, we are cradled.

Even though a child may have terrible experiences early in life, the unconscious power of the womb experience cannot be shaken— but is often not tapped. When we learn to help others discover ways to nurture themselves, and find nurture, we get in touch with that well of strength and fulfillment within ourselves. It is a spring which flows from deep within.

Since I have no arms, for a part of my early years I yearned for arms with which to care for myself. While compensating, the feeling remained.

One day, I discovered an old scripture for the first time—and the well gushed forth: *The eternal God is thy refuge, and underneath are the everlasting arms* (Deuteronomy 33:27). Those loving, nurturing arms were there all along! And from that day, I felt that sea of support. The supporting love of God remains all around us from our very beginning, much of it unconscious, often when we are not aware of his presence.

- *Discover your self-worth. Encourage it in others.*

In this discovery religion is powerfully import. In religion, we recognize an ultimate expression of self-worth. Medicine cannot quite express it. Medical science can point out the importance of community acceptance of the individual, the need for self-esteem and personhood. But in religion we have the opportunity of saying that from the holy books of our basic religions—that at the very basis of the universe, God cares for you. You are a cared-for and beloved person!

People respond to persons with disabilities in terms of that person's own sense of self-worth. The aura which comes from a person's assurance of being accepted, of being whole, shines through to the other. Spiritual care is a critically important, potent ally in the rehabilitation process.

- *The religious community must bless and empower persons with disabilities.*

I have been ordained for over half a century. I was made a minister in my denomination, even though I didn't fit the usual categories. After all, isn't a minister someone who from the pulpit raises his arms and pounds the pulpit? Yet the congregation said, "We believe that you have gifts and abilities more than that. We will indeed ordain you!"

"How will Wilke perform the sacraments—to baptize those he brings to faith?"

For the service of baptism the minister stands at the baptismal font, an ornately carved column with a silver bowl at the top for the baptismal water. At the appointed time, she dips her fingers into the bowl and sprinkles a few drops of water onto the forehead and cheek of the child.

Having no fingers, I had to improvise.

The words of the baptismal ritual pronounced, I stand before family and congregation. Then I kiss the surface of the water in the font and immediately kiss the child's forehead. Enough water adheres to my lips to allow the ecclesiastically proper three drops to course gently down the forehead of the child. Then I go on with the prayers.

- *The religious community must then take the lead in becoming welcoming and inclusive to persons with disabilities.*

All persons must share congregational leadership. Ordain, bless, empower their abilities. Become community one to another.

Caring about another person is never easy, but always worth the investment.

Loving parents saw my innate abilities long before I realized my limitations (and we all have them!). Equally, communities of faith must nurture the God-given, inborn abilities of all its members.

- *Promote peace and harmony wherever you can.*

Don't skip past the depth of this statement! Preventing war reduces one cause of disability. Rehabilitation became an institutional force *after* thousands of wounded soldiers returned from battle, bodies misshapen and torn. We must defend our country against harm, to be sure; but the seeds of destruction remain long after war ends. In Mid-East deserts, children will for a generation pick up mines planted by their own side, and by Americans, or by the United Nations' allied forces and have a hand or leg blown off. A whole *next* generation of people suddenly become involved.

Ironically, most people assume that it was Canada and the United States which led in the creation of the United Nations' International Year of Disabled Persons. Be surprised when I tell you that the source initiating that movement was Muammar Quadhafi. Quadhafi! He led in creating the UN proposal because so many children in the Libyan deserts were picking up mines left there from a generation before, planted during World War II. He then petitioned the UN to develop a new dedication to rehabilitative efforts worldwide.

- *Faith communities which do not have within them the active presence and participation of persons with disabilities are themselves dis-abled.*

The Vatican, Rome, 1993. The Pope's invitation came to me and two dozen others to speak at the Catholic Church's conference on ministry and persons with disabilities. The Holy Father's words crossed many boundaries, applying to both clergy and health professionals: "We in the religious community need to recognize, more fully than ever, the place which religion has in the physical and inner healing of persons who have disabilities." I would add to that: persons with disabilities have a place in the religious community. Without their presence, the community of faith is not only incomplete: it is *dis*-membered.

All leaders in our society, representing varied professional backgrounds and secular activities, need to recognize that what the Pope is doing from the religious community's side, all need to do from their vocational placements, including physical medicine and rehabilitation.

- *Religion and faith are allies of the healing process.*

More than that! Hope is the balm of broken souls, faith the grounding.

All too often, spiritual resources are kept at bay in the medical process. Faith itself is not necessarily religious, but it is always spiritual. Faith is an attitude about one's life, and the life around us. Without faith in the goodness and nurturing of those around us, we cannot survive—much less heal.

This is the metaphor for medical care. Divest health care of spiritual healing, and healing diminishes. For some persons, it will disappear.

- ***The medical community should see not just the presenting circumstance, but the whole person.***

During World War II, Dr. Henry Kessler invited me to San Francisco, where he was then Captain Kessler in the orthopedic wards. In the course of my "TDY" (temporary duty), we became fast friends. We saw in each other the kind of hopes we held for rehabilitation medicine—that the discipline would recognize the place of spiritual care in the healing process.

At the end of that week, Dr. Kessler said, "Harold, as soon as this war is over, I want you to come to the Kessler Institute. Let me fit you with prosthetic arms."

After the war was over, he did indeed invite me to speak to staff and patients. At the end of a few days, he said, "Harold, I've changed my mind about your situation. Fitting you with prosthetic arms would provide me with professional satisfaction, but it wouldn't really help *you* that much. You're fully independent just as you learned it yourself!"

Some years later, we met again at a conference in Sydney, Australia.

"Henry," I said, "do you remember the time I told you that those of us in ministry don't have the little black bag you have in medicine? That symbol of authority and ability."

Dr. Kessler smiled. "Harold, you don't need the little black bag. For that matter, you don't need the little black book (Bible). You have the ability—it's right in you." He added, "It's in me, too. It's in our *personhood.*"

- ***Persons with disabilities can fill normal jobs.***

Employers, fill those jobs! Our society now acknowledges that persons with disabilities are productive and capable in the work force. The creative contributions of such persons has only begun to be mined. For example, did you know that one of the most useful and universally used of all inventions—velcro—was designed by a person with a disability?

Persons with disabilities are also leaders in the work place. You the reader can probably name several, both personally and publicly known. Others wait for opportunities to add their own gifts and talents for a more productive society.

- **In rehabilitation and health care settings, remember
  that the person (sometimes referred to as patient) is
  at the center of the therapeutic team.**

Tact prevents me from decrying the doublespeak rampant in modern healthcare. You've heard the various mutations of this principle: quality care; quality assurance; do more with less. All of these words describe the system, the structure.

The person is the bottom line. Any organization reworking this equation will have short-term success and eventually disappear in the long term.

- **If we can love: this is the touchstone. If we are able to help
  the other person receive love and to offer love, we will have
  healed them.**

These words of Karl Menninger ring strong and true. Love is that quality of caring which goes far beyond professional expertise. The healing power of love should not be underestimated either.

- **All aspects of life are open to a person with a disability.**

But, you say—there's so much that people with disabilities cannot do.

Then again, who can do everything? Look instead at how much you've got. Live in hope, not fear.

My eldest child Bill, now a nuclear physicist in Cambridge, was born three years after Peg and I were married. At that time, we searched the medical data about what would happen if a congenitally limbless person (myself) had a child with a "normal person," as is my wife.

"What will happen? Will our baby be born without arms, like me?" There was little information for us. Believing things would be all right, we went ahead with hope. And Bill, who is normal (except that he's a Ph.D. and a nuclear physicist) is the "normal" result of our decision to have a child. The same is true for all five of our sons.

I am deeply blessed to hear my congenitally limbless friends from the thalidomide tragedy report, "Our first child was born normal; we are relieved." And later: "Our second child was recently born normal; everything is fine."

CONCLUSION: IMAGINE MORE!

I offer these principles to the reader, which arise from my half-century of work in the rehabilitation field alongside my chosen field of ministry. They are but a distillation of learnings which continue even today.

I close with a story from my earliest years.

My mother, soon after my birth, took me along to the grocery store. Someone in the store turned to my mother and said, "Your baby?" pointing to the swaddled object on her arm. My mother said "Yes." And the woman said, "I heard the church bells this morning tolling the death of an infant, and I hoped that it was your poor little baby."

This reaction may strike a memory for readers whose disability is congenital. I hope that their parental response was the strong one that my mother gave: "No," she said, "life is better."

Only a year or two later, my mother was able to demonstrate this learning for me. I was sitting on the floor in the bedroom trying to put on my shirt. My mother had opened up the shirt and placed it on the floor, on a pillow. I was trying to get it on over my head and shoulders, then down over my side. It was difficult! My mother stood there and watched me. I repeat, she stood and watched me. Not one hand, not one finger did she lift to do it for me. She saw how frustrated I was; but she lifted not one finger to help!

Her friend stood beside, aghast. "Ida, why don't you help that child!"

And my mother said, "I am helping him."

Helping by not helping is difficult for parents and professionals, all of us. Allowing the individual to do it his or her own way, different from our own, independently—this is difficult indeed.

I was lucky to have that kind of parental—and through my life, professional—caring. We are called to help persons develop within themselves the resources which are theirs, and to call upon those resources. A world full of opportunity and wonder is then opened.

EDITOR'S NOTE

To further explore the course of Wilke's career and its influence on the field of religion and disability, see the article included in this volume written by Robert Pietsch.

Who Will Move the Next Mountain?
Congregational Hospitality
and Community Involvement

William A. Blair, DMin
Dana Davidson Blair, MS, RN

SUMMARY. *Section I* voices concern about traditional attitudes among the religious community regarding persons with disabilities. Such attitudes have hindered commitment to awareness, acceptance, and inclusion. It discusses religion's unique potential in the advocacy of quality of life and dignity.

Section II offers practical suggestions for community and congregational partnership in becoming more welcoming and inclusive to persons with disabilities. *[Article copies available from The Haworth Document Delivery Service: 1-800-342-9678. E-mail address: getinfo@haworth.com]*

KEYWORDS. Religion and disability, advocacy, dignity, civic responsibility, inclusion

Bill Gaventa's article in this volume illuminates the movement of health care chaplaincy from institutional to community settings. In this article, we will clarify why it is critical for community organizations to assist communities of faith in their efforts to include

William A. Blair and Dana Davidson Blair are Co-Editors of the *Journal of Religion in Disability & Rehabilitation.*

[Haworth co-indexing entry note]: "Who Will Move the Next Mountain? Congregational Hospitality and Community Involvement." Blair, William A., and Dana Davidson Blair. Co-published simultaneously in *Journal of Religion in Disability & Rehabilitation* (The Haworth Press, Inc.) Vol. 2, No. 4, 1996, pp. 81-90; and: *A Look Back: The Birth of the Americans with Disabilities Act* (ed: Robert C. Anderson) The Haworth Press, Inc., 1996, pp. 81-90. Single or multiple copies of this article are available from The Haworth Document Delivery Service [1-800-342-9678, 9:00 a.m. - 5:00 p.m. (EST). E-mail address: getinfo@haworth.com].

persons with disabilities. The religious community has great potential to lead in advocacy and social inclusion for persons with disabilities. To achieve this goal, congregations must redefine and strengthen their commitment to families and people who experience disability.

I. THE ROLE AND RESPONSIBILITY OF FAITH COMMUNITIES

Background

For the more than 43 million people with disabilities in the United States, society has become more accessible since the passage of the Americans with Disabilities Act (ADA). But most of them would agree that the widespread, open-hearted changes that the Act was meant to inspire have yet to be realized. *The ADA's goals may never be realized if the support of organized religion does not grow.* With policies on paper and the ramps in place, there is a tendency for communities of faith to become content. We congratulate ourselves on what has been achieved, while there is a very real need for our congregations to step forward into a role of advocacy for the human rights of people with disabilities.

Historically, those who experienced disability had a shorter life expectancy than today. Many often succumbed to massive infections, accidents and the effects of neglect. Modern medicine, while it has not always been able to cure, has developed treatments which prolong life. As medical technology becomes more sophisticated and effective, the number of people who survive disabling injury and disease increases. We can therefore expect the number of persons with disabilities in our society to remain high.

The ADA provides a starting point for social inclusion and improved quality of life for persons experiencing disability. This law embraces a basic social morality that religion might have taught (and which some religions *have* taught) all along. Changes have been gradual and mostly in terms of physical access (ramps, etc.) to ensure compliance with the law. Inclusion, acceptance and welcoming attitudes cannot be legislated and will take much longer, for these are relationship issues.

Medical rehabilitation professionals are not the only ones responsible for quality of life for persons with disabilities. This responsibility must be matched and led by the religious community. What other social force can bring such sweeping enlightenment to our local neighborhoods and cities? The lead must be made by clear-eyed persons of faith, those who have an understanding of ethics and morals. Communities of faith certainly come to mind in this regard. The greater part of our country's population still listens when religion speaks. It is time to teach the truth about people with disabilities as we purge the old myths and traditions. Such attitudes have made so many communities of faith inaccessible and unwelcoming in the past.

The inclination to stereotype is strong in American society. There is hardly any group that has not suffered the effects of categorization at one time or another. Stereotypes isolate people from one another. In the past, religious stereotypes have identified people with disabilities as "cursed," both saints and sinners, the "despised of God," and much more.

How has our society come to view people with disabilities in this way? Why do the non-disabled pity and exclude persons with disabilities?

Our country's system of beliefs bear the heavy influence of Hebrew, Greek and Christian tenets. Religious belief often nurtures the view that disability is the result of sin and is both a punishment and means of atonement, even spiritual purification. Greek tradition gave us the perception that persons with disabilities are abhorrent, inferior people whom society need not consider unless they can improve or recover. The practical, secular view perceives misfortune as a natural occurrence, assuming that behaviors have consequences. Under this view, certain disabilities are regarded as elements of life that can be controlled to some extent.

American society has developed and taught our children some form of these traditional thoughts. It is unfortunate that these traditional views emphasize the *cause* of disability. We ask "why" disability happens, as though the question can tell us something vital about human suffering. It does not. God's assurances of love for us, in both the Old and New Testaments, are very clear and often repeated.

The Bible instructs us to behave toward others as we wish them to behave toward us. Part of religion's purpose in our lives is to guide us toward empathy, teach us to ask ourselves how we, in the shoes of any person who has suffered, would want to be perceived by society. Would we want to struggle simply to move through an average day in a world that is not designed for us? Would we want to be left out of so much of what makes life agreeable and fun? Would we want to be perceived as dirty, incompetent and less valued? Fair treatment and just living are reciprocal. *We* must be the cause and the source of changing our world into one of acceptance, inclusion and access, a world that leaves judgment to God.

One great loss (among many losses experienced by persons with disabilities and their families) is the nearly automatic forfeiture of dignity. People with disabilities often feel that their presence in society has diminished, that the respect one human shows another is not considered relevant in their lives. Dignity is a basic need, something we vastly prefer to pity or even honest compassion. It is a need that encompasses many others, and it exists in the soul of every person who is somehow "different." The heart of religion is the dignity of human life. One of religion's higher designs is the development of spiritual values that honor human life as God's creation. It is not religion's task or privilege to judge *which* life is valuable, but only to celebrate life as a gift from God and therefore to dignify each life.

In the practice of religion, however, it has somehow become more comfortable to assume that only some of us are actually the beloved children of God, i.e., those who are in no way "different." Or we find some other extreme—whatever relieves the conscience. We are not visibly neglectful: we build the ramps, provide the interpreters, install the handrails. We invest money, but not the spirit of the faith community. The proper motions are made, but the welcome is no better than what one might find in a hotel that installs an extra towel rack and calls it a handrail. If religion's welcome is weak, the rest of society feels no obligation to make more than token gestures of accessibility. If religion feels no outrage, no despair over the lack of inclusion and the devaluation of life people with disabilities encounter, why should the secular world involve itself in advocacy for their rights or treat them with dignity?

Ramps, handrails, elevators and wide doorways make buildings—but not necessarily hearts—accessible. One church, synagogue or mosque per community practicing genuine acceptance is commendable, but it is not enough.

Congregations: The Heart of Community Care

Consider this scenario, one decade from now:

Millions of baby boomers reach retirement. Medicare has long since been reduced to little more than a supplement in total health costs. Social security faces extinction.

With these aging millions comes the incidence of age-related disability, the likes of which our society has never seen. Families struggle to care for their elderly, who often equal or outpace the number of children born to them. Single-parent families add to the dilemma; the need for emotional and practical support is at critical mass.

To whom will these persons and families turn when in the throes of personal crisis, pain and chaos?

Only a few ministers and their congregations have yet to realize the community need brewing on their doorstep. The enlightened ones are wisely planning now so as to better minister to their communities in caring, compassionate and responsible ways.

II. PRACTICAL SUGGESTIONS FOR CONGREGATIONAL AND COMMUNITY PARTNERSHIP

Congregational Responses

Respite Care Teams/Programs. Respite care provides relief to full-time caregivers. The makeup and structure of such ministries reflect the diversity and needs of each congregation. For example, one congregation in Pelham, Alabama set up a program where parents can bring their children with disabilities, and their able-bodied siblings, to the congregation on Friday nights. Trained volunteers involve the children in an evening of fun activities while the parents go out. For full-time parental caregivers, this is indeed a luxury.

Other respite care ministries become programs unto themselves which serve persons beyond the congregation. Trained laypersons make home visits, provide transportation to medical appointments, and other caring interventions. Through these contacts, connections with the person's worship community are maintained or even strengthened.

Congregational Care Teams are composed of both the able-bodied and persons with disabilities. Together, they provide ministry and care to fellow members in need. Such relational ministries represent congregational mainstreaming at its best. For too long, the religious community has held a caretaking role toward persons with disabilities. When attitudes and relationships are broadened, persons with disabilities become leaders within each congregation. All persons have gifts, talents and abilities to offer their community of faith.

Ministers will increasingly appreciate lay involvement in their congregation's life.

Community Partnerships

Health care reform is concerned for its own survival, and its impact is catalyzing dramatic changes within the community. The new cutting edge for community involvement rests in responsible, forward-thinking partnerships between organizations, the disability community and the largest single demographic segment of our society: the religious community.

One of the clearest and most visionary expressions of such partnership is the creation of local or state-based community programs which unite these social resources. For example, the Lakeshore Foundation (Birmingham, Alabama) has established a local/state based *Religion and Disability Program* to stimulate the religious community's involvement with persons who have disabilities. Lakeshore Foundation—a nonprofit operating organization—is not affiliated with any religious group. Their concern and vision rests in a keen understanding of the need to provide an array of services to improve the lives of persons with disabilities.

They accomplish this mission through a variety of integrated programs. The Lakeshore Foundation's internationally recognized wheelchair sports program provides opportunities for both the competitive and recreational athlete. Program components include (among others) *Super Sports* for children and youth, *Outdoor Adventure*, and *SportsQuest* which promotes fitness and wellness. *Lakeshore's Religion and Disability Program* assists faith communities in their efforts to become more welcoming and inclusive to persons with disabilities. The program is directed by a clinically trained chaplain with experience in the field of disability.

Many congregations desire to welcome and include persons with disabilities, yet need guidance and practical resources. Likewise, persons with disabilities want and deserve to participate in the rights and obligations of their faith—but often cannot even get into the congregation. Once inside, they often feel isolated and less than welcome. Lakeshore Foundation's state-based *Religion and Disability* program provides training, education and resources for congregations desiring to become more welcoming and inclusive.

Programs such as these recognize and actively promote inclusion. People with disabilities deserve to participate actively and fully in the life of their communities.

Becoming Responsible Faith Communities

Securing Congregational Training About Disability. Clergy who have limited training or exposure to disability should seek out experienced others to assist their congregations. For example, many areas have access to clinically trained chaplains who serve at rehabilitation or other disability service organizations. That professional might help the congregation strategize ways to create awareness of disability for members of that faith community.

An excellent beginning point is to conduct a "Disability Awareness Day" held on your congregation's regular Sabbath service. Persons with disabilities lead in the liturgy, prayers and sermons. After that event has been conducted, congregations are generally receptive to more focused events such as special emphasis studies on a weeknight or sabbath evening. Further training opportunities can then be carried out based on that congregation's needs and ministry goals.

Congregational Hospitality. When we invite a guest into our home, much planning and care occur long before the person arrives. Consideration is given to our guests' comfort, special needs or interests, and putting them at ease. In short, the person feels welcome and included. Inclusive congregations attract people who don't mind giving and working for their faith community because they want others to experience that kind of caring environment too.

Hospitality especially applies to the religious community. Ramps are important—but they are not enough. Once inside, we must help all persons feel welcomed and included. Attitudes are more difficult to modify than buildings, but the long-term benefit for all persons is greater. Congregations benefit when they provide hospitality training to their ushers, leaders, and members in general.

Accessibility Considerations. Buildings convey messages about a faith community. A house of worship that is visibly accessible from its entrance creates an immediate impression to all persons that they are welcomed and included. When making modifications (or planning for new construction), consult with persons who have disabilities. In spite of good intentions, able-bodied planners do not possess personal experience as a guide for creating the atmosphere for hospitality.

Relationships and Attitudinal Considerations. Relationships are the most important area for progress—or distance—regarding inclusion. There are no glib or immediate remedies to correct how people relate with each other, whether through lack of experience or ingrained cultural attitudes. Congregations cannot always respond immediately—structural modifications are sometimes beyond the financial means of smaller faith communities. However, this should not be an excuse for responding sensitively and with hospitality in other ways. One can always reach out through relationships, which are the most enduring of all forms of support and care.

CONCLUSION

This volume's theme remembers the dedicated efforts of many advocates who helped bring about passage of the Americans with Disabilities Act (ADA) of 1990. In this achievement, there are numerous champions whose names will never be recorded, yet their contributions remain an enduring legacy to millions of Americans and their descendants.

This book also poses a summons to the religious community,

which has not always been enthusiastic in supporting the societal goals embodied in the ADA. Local congregations (and their denominational bodies) are not legally required to comply with the ADA's inclusive goals. However, the religious community does have a moral mandate to lead in welcoming and including persons with disabilities. And people of faith must answer to a far higher power. The religious community has leaders who can strengthen our calling to include *all* people in this way.

Every generation should have a Harold Wilke, a voice both spiritual and practical that speaks from a heart made courageous by strong convictions. Dr. Wilke's talents as a writer are considerable. Even stronger than his words has been his life, an example of faith and determination, of selfless giving of himself for the benefit of all. He has lived what he believes.

Dr. Wilke has made a difference in the lives of a great many people, but perhaps his most valuable contribution to our lives has been hope. He accentuates the positive and stands with great dignity when others say "No" through their attitudes. He has taught us to think in terms of possibilities and to pursue what seems impossible. Dr. Wilke's life exemplifies what it means to have the strength of an active religious faith; his actions reveal what congregations—meaning the people in them—can become. Faith translated into deeds is a living testament to the power of God. Mountains have been moved.

The move toward inclusion and equity is still very new, still in need of strong support. We cannot depend entirely on the ADA to open the doors that remain closed to people with disabilities—laws do not open hearts or minds, nor is their business to teach decency. Those responsibilities are within the domain of religion.

Religion's strength already extends into the community and shares common ground with rehabilitation. The religious community has the potential to sustain what has been achieved and to accomplish much more. The question is, does organized religion want to go beyond myth and superstition toward understanding and acceptance—does it even see the mountain that must be moved?

RECOMMENDED READINGS

Brightman, Alan J., ed. *Ordinary Moments: The Disabled Experience*. Baltimore: University Park Press, 1984. *Softcover, 160 pp.*

Eisland, Nancy. *The Disabled God: Toward a Liberatory Theology of Disability*. Nashville: Abingdon, 1994. *Softcover, 139 pp.*

Govig, Stewart D. *Strong at the Broken Places: Persons with Disabilities and the Church*. Louisville: Westminster/John Knox Press, 1989. *Softcover, 145 pp.*

Merrick, Lewis H., ed. *And Show Steadfast Love: A Theological Look at Grace, Hospitality, Disabilities, and the Church*. Louisville: Presbyterian Publishing House, 1993. *Softcover, 102 pp.*

Murphy, Judith K. *Sharing Care: The Christian Ministry of Respite Care*. New York: United Church Press, 1986. *Softcover, 58 pp.*

Webb-Mitchell, Brett. *God Plays Piano, Too: The Spiritual Lives of Disabled Children*. New York: Crossroad Publishers, 1993. *Hardcover, 200 pp.*

Wilke, Harold H. *Creating the Caring Congregation*. Nashville: Abingdon, 1980. *Softcover, 110 pp.*